THE PLANT POWERED PENIS

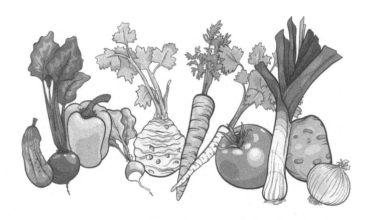

THE PLANT POWERED PENIS

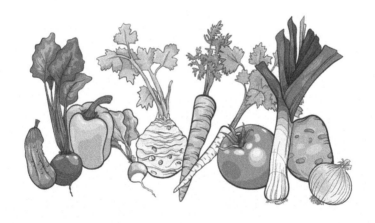

MINDY MYLREA

COPYRIGHT

DISCLAIMER

This book is not intended as a substitute for the medical advice of physicians. The reader should regularly consult a physician in matters relating to his/her health and particularly with respect to any symptoms that may require diagnosis or medical attention.

REVIEWS

Foods have powerful effects on health—they can help you lose weight, lower cholesterol, and even reduce your cancer risk. But there is one benefit you might not have anticipated, and that is their effect on your sex life. Give it a try, and you'll see what I mean. This engaging book brings you the information you need, along with delicious recipes to put it to work.

Neal D. Barnard, MD
Adjunct Professor
George Washington University School of Medicine
President, Physicians Committee

This entertaining book engages readers with the science and research of eating a whole food, plant-based diet without added oil and also with Mindy's personal experience of how plant-based nutrition plays an important role in a healthy marriage/partnership and health overall.

John McDougall, MD
Founder of the McDougall Program
Best-selling author—The Starch Solution

Playful and sexy in its delivery, the information Mylrea shares is health positive regardless of your genitalia. Whether you choose to go fully vegan or not, a plant-based diet is clearly associated with enhanced wellbeing, reducing the risk of chronic illness such as obesity, diabetes, heart disease, and cancer. Helpful motivating tips and enticing recipes provide practical resources to encourage the adoption of improved nutrition for a healthier lifestyle.

Donald I. Abrams, MD, Integrative Oncologist,
UCSF Osher Center for Integrative Medicine
Professor of Clinical Medicine,
University of California San Francisco

IT'S ABOUT TIME for this book to come out! I've health coached hundreds of men over a decade now, and they need this NOW more than ever! This quick, easy-to-read guide will give you all the "action" steps you need to take your health back into your own hands! Thank you, Mindy, for bringing this book to life! Can't wait to give them out as Holiday Gifts!

Michelle Joy Kramer
Board Certified Health Coach,
CHHC, AADP

Vegan is the new viagra! In this delightful book you'll learn that what's good for your heart is good for all of your organs. Why take a blue pill when you can eat a green leaf?

Chef AJ
Author: *The Secrets To Ultimate Weight Loss*

Books on sex and diet are among the most popular books read today. This is a book about both. It is a must-read for every man that wants to maintain a healthy body and a healthy sex life throughout his life. This book demonstrates how the power of plant-based nutrition can help men maintain a healthy sex life throughout life.

John Westerdahl, PhD, MPH, RDN, FAND
Radio Talk Show Host
Past Chair, Vegetarian Nutrition
Dietetic Practice Group of the
Academy of Nutrition and Dietetics

What a great read. Informative, hopeful, hilarious, and full of tangible action items to include right away to support optimal health. The lessons in this book will help every gender and every cell and organ in your body."

— Ocean Robbins, Co-founder
Food Revolution Network
Author, 31-Day Food Revolution

DEDICATION

This book is dedicated to my husband, Bruce. Without him guiding my way, censoring me where needed, and loving me more than I could have ever hoped for in life, this book would not have been written. I cannot begin to put into words how much I love this man. So, I will leave it at that.

~ ~ ~

EPIGRAPH

Plants protect the penis.

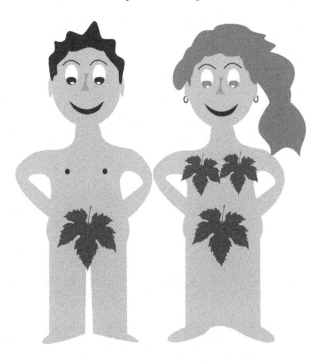

— Mindy Mylrea

~

PREFACE

I hope you find this book light hearted, fun, informative, and inspiring. In all my years of teaching I have learned that the subject matter only comes to life when you, the teacher, bring it to life. So I hope I brought to light an otherwise limp topic. I hope that you have a deep appreciation for the penis, for the men who own them, and for the women who hang out with them.

— Mindy Mylrea

ACKNOWLEDGEMENTS

I want to acknowledge and pay tribute to my miraculous husband, Bruce. First for unselfishly providing me with almost 40 years of amazing erections and allowing me to write about it, and second, for dedicating his life to sharing his story and his vast knowledge in the relationship of food with health and what we can do to affect our outcomes and to live not a normal life but an optimal life. I met Bruce when I was only 21 and fell in love with him that moment, and our love for each other has only grown. When Bruce was diagnosed with advanced-stage prostate cancer short of ten years ago, we both were blindsided. We had no emotional tools to deal with this earthquake in our lives. Over the past nine years, we have dealt with many ups and downs and have always come out the other end with a new tool to add to our emotional tool box. Cancer sucks, but how you deal with it can suck even worse. Bruce is a fighter, and he has taken his new, sometimes very difficult life and created a mission to help others with the tools that we never had before. The new normal has become men having ED, then CVD or diabetes, living the last ten years of life compromised, and then dying an early death. If this book can help in any way that their normal transforms to optimal then I have done what I set out to do.

Thanks to my three amazing sons Drew, Chris, and Casey who put up with all their mom's crazy shenanigans and aren't too embarrassed by their mom's desire and delight to talk penis whenever possible. I love you so much.

Thanks to Dr. T. Colin Campbell for leading the charge and writing the ground-breaking book, *The China Study*. This book transformed my sceptic carnivore husband into a plant loving herbivore and mapped the trajectory of our careers for the past ten years.

Thanks to Dr. Michael Greger whose counsel has steered us to create our nonprofit One Day to Wellness and who selflessly provides research and science-based information for all of us to understand.

Thanks to both my cover artist, Lauren Katz, and my editor, Grace Michael, for their time and amazing talent making my book look so good outside and in. Without their expertise, this book would be coming to you on the back of a napkin.

Thanks to all of you who are reading this book. I hope it helps your normal transform to optimal.

CONTENTS

INTRODUCTION

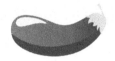

It's not hard to make decisions once you know what your values are.

— Roy E. Disney

One to change a few. A few to change many. Many to change the world. Starts with one.

— Anonymous

Why am I writing this book? I don't even own a penis!

I am excited to write this book and have you read it and then have you leave it on a bus so someone else can read it. It is true that I don't own a penis. However, I know a lot of men who do and my love for these men runs deep. It is my duty to assist in the safe keeping of the erection, and this is why I have to share this information with you. I am not a doctor nor am I a scientist, but I am a damn good researcher, and I am a great cook (recipes to prove it provided). I only have included in this book what evidence and science points to as the best foods to eat every day for health and vitality.

My goal is to honor all those men and their penises and all the women who love them.

Sprinkled throughout the book are my penis tips. Each of these starts with my own personal penis perspective and then are validated with research, science, and fun bits of information corresponding with my personal insights or stories. These are appropriately titled "Tip About the Tip." This provides a collaboration of my vast penis knowledge and then the research to support the tip.

THE PROUD PENIS

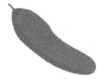

It is what it is.

— Anonymous

There is one thing I know for sure. Men love their penises. From the moment they are born, they know there is something awesome down there and that it needs to be protected. Even though their penis isn't going anywhere, there is a need to keep checking multiple times a day that that magic wand is indeed still there. The phenomena that men (and I am including all ages here) have to just hold their penis is so strange to me. Go into my house any afternoon when I was growing up and you would witness my three brothers all lined up on the couch watching a random TV show and where would at least one hand be? Yup—in the pants. Not in a sexual way, but just a nonchalant hand down the pants to make sure all was copacetic way. Geez, you know. Everything was hanging right; all was in its place, and everything was still there.

I went on to have three boys of my own. All with penises and all with the same fondness of hands down the pants while relaxing on the couch just because. Because we were very open with our boys about sexuality, they were in turn not shy around the house. Let's just say penises were popping out from every corner. Yes, just because.

I got to experience, for better or worse, just how proud boys are of what their penises can actually do. Erect penises can hold a towel all by themselves on the way to the shower, their stream can sink any object in the toilet over and over again. And unfortunately, they can get caught in zipper after zipper—this is where mom came to the rescue or mom was the culprit. The other great feats of the penis I just watched from afar rolling my eyes. Girls. Why didn't I make girls?

According to an article written by Cosmo Frank for Cosmopolitan magazine titled, "11 Things Guys Secretly Do with Their Penises (March 31, 2015)."

> **Just hold it, ever so gently.** All the time. Just walking around the house doing chores and holding our penis. Holding our penis while driving (not illegal). Pretty much anything we can do with one hand, we'll use the other hand to hold our penis.

This is what I know is true. Men love their penises, and I am a woman that happens to love them too. I want every man to have the opportunity to not only make sure it is still there, but to be able to use it to its fullest capacity. Eating plants make for a Proud Penis—one that stands to attention when called upon ready for action at a moment's notice. So, let's get to it men. Let's go out there and hunt for the foods that will stiffen the loins and harness the woodie.

THE POWER OF Ps

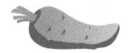

The Gods created certain kinds of beings to replenish our bodies; they are the trees and the plants and the seeds.

— Plato

My loving, highly sexually-functioning husband of 40 years was diagnosed with advanced prostate cancer nine years ago. Up until that point, sex was a given. We didn't ever think that perhaps someday his sexual function might diminish. It never crossed our minds that one day we would be told by his doctors that Bruce would quickly decline sexually because of his cancer treatments and that we should prepare ourselves for a life of little to no erectile function, low to no sex drive, and life as we had known it for going on 40 years would be altered dramatically forever.

A funny thing about that—sex between my husband and myself has never been better. All that I had read was wrong. The doctors were wrong. And I was wrong to believe that we were a statistic and that all men with advanced prostate cancer have the same symptoms and outcomes. Bruce has endured a prostatectomy (the removal of the prostate) and two rounds of hormone treatment. Hormone treatment is basically shutting off the testosterone in the body. Bruce says that he has been through menopause twice. He has had two rounds of radiation and one round of chemotherapy. All along the way, we have lived battling the emotional roller coaster of monthly blood tests with rising and then lowering and then rising again PSA (Prostate Specific Antigen). PSA is the marker for prostate cancer—this number should be zero without a prostate. Rising PSA numbers without a prostate most likely means that the prostate cancer has spread to somewhere else in his body.

This cancer story is what we live with every day. What we don't live with are the crummy statistics. Bruce has taken matters into his own hands and mounted a defense with mindful eating, stress reduction, living with passion and purpose, and not giving in. Too many men thinking that ED is just something that happens acquiesce and accept the inevitable without a fight. But what if the inevitable wasn't inevitable? What if you had more control than you thought you did? What if what you hear and read doesn't take into account the most important piece of the puzzle—You. You are unique and not a stat, and the choices you make have everything to do with the outcomes you end up with. Bruce is living proof that stats are only stats and the individual has a whole lot to do with how the story plays out.

If you are going through health challenges, you are not alone in this journey, and with the right information, the side effects of treatments and outcome can be minimized.

How in the world, with all the treatments Bruce has gone through, has he been able to have even one erection let alone having them on a daily basis? I attribute this to three factors:

The Power of Plants

As you have probably guessed by the title of this book, incorporating plants into one's diet every day is the focus, highlighting fruits, veggies, whole grains, and legumes. The benefits (as Bruce and I call them), and how to integrate them, is with a "lean to the green." Spoiler alert. If the vast amount of research between the relationship of diet and ED (and for that matter CVD, certain types of cancer, diabetes, and other chronic diseases) showed that eating animal products supported blood flow to the groin, it would be included. But even if you do see research touting the benefits of an animal-based diet you have to look at who funded the study, how many people participated in the study, what was the duration of the study, and how many other studies support the claim? These studies are just not there.

I will outline the research to date on vascular blood flow as it relates to nutrition and the plant powered food we eat every day that supports the pipes. Achieving and then keeping an erection all boils down to blood flow. I will share with you the importance and starring role of what you eat has to do with how you feel about yourself and how your body performs at its best. You will learn about specific foods to eat every day to increase blood flow for every aspect of your life—not only your sex life.

The Power of Purpose

When Bruce was diagnosed with prostate cancer, our world turned upside down. Up until that point we were impervious to emotional upheaval. We had skated along for our entire married life basically unscathed. No rocky times in our marriage, three well-adjusted children that had gone on to find their way and most importantly find their way off mom and dad's payroll. Life was good, or so we thought. What we had no way of knowing was that, inside Bruce's body, he was watering the seeds of prostate cancer every day for who knows how long and the outcome was not good.

When faced with a life -threating prognosis, what's a couple to do? Lay down and feel sorry for ourselves (we did do our share of that) or find out everything we could about what we needed to do to take control of the situation? Our journey started with listening and following blindly, but we soon turned that ship around to understanding we had more control than we thought we did on everything from side effects to treatment to outcome, and most important to mindset.

10

We realized that our path was our own to make, and we had to arm ourselves with knowledge and information that even the doctors weren't well versed in. Hence here is where the purpose comes in. Shortly after Bruce was diagnosed and shortly after learning the truth that the choices we make have a huge impact on our outcome, we became totally committed to sharing our knowledge with others.

Being on the speaking circuit already for so many years lecturing on fitness and general wellness, we became laser focused on nutrition and its relationship to all that is health and well-being. We came to understand that the traditionally trained doctor does not get any or very little nutritional education in medical school. And being that poor nutrition is one of the leading causes of disease in this country, this unbiased, science-based, and most importantly—not-for-profit information had to be shared.

Aligning ourselves with powerful other nonprofits who also believe in the truth without industry influence (see resource section), Bruce and I have found our true purpose, and it is with this purpose that we are energized beyond measure. Talk about a libido booster. Having a purpose ignites the flame and stokes the fire in every sense of the word.

Bruce and I are living our passion traveling worldwide in a fruit and veggie covered RV leading our "One Day to Wellness" and "Cooking and Coaching" programs. Doing what you know is right and inhaling it in with every breath brings life and meaning to everything else in your life.

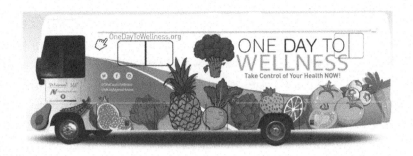

The Power of Partnership

Your sexual partner plays a huge role in the intricate intimacy dance, as I call it, that marks true sexual satisfaction. I am not talking about casual sex (just for fun with no emoional commitment), utilitarian sex (the sex that takes place in the early AM just so that the early morning erection will subside so

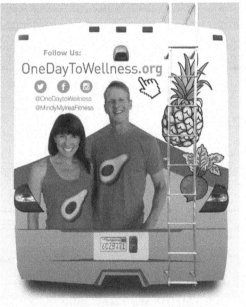

that aiming in the toilet is possible), or masturbation sex that can be mastered anytime and anywhere no matter what. Actually, masturbation, as you will learn later, has been shown to enhance marital satisfaction. I am not in any way insinuating that these sexual interprettations cannot be important in a man or women's life. I am just pointing out that erectile function interacts with the emotional as well as the physical dance couples play, and keeping this part of the relationship running smoothly is a very important part of the dance.

Intimacy between two people who have chosen to come together in every sense of the word is magic. There is no better aphrodisiac than to totally surrender to the other emotionally and physically. There is something pretty amazing about the connection of foreplay and outcome, and I am going to propose to you that foreplay begins in the grocery store, then the kitchen. Then and only then in the bedroom. The connection with what foods we chose to buy, cook, and eat together lays the ground work for all that follows. Plant seeds, water, and nurture, then eat those seeds and your garden will flourish. Your relationship works in the exact same way. Only in this book you will learn that the plants you grow in your garden fuel your emotional and sexual health.

If you are a woman reading this book, know that just like Lainie Kazan who played Toula's mother, Maria Portokalos, in *My Big Fat Greek Wedding* proclaimed, "Let me tell you something, Toula: The man is the head, but the woman is the neck, and she can turn the head any way she wants." Women have tremendous influence, and our choices affect those around us. When you eat with intention and mindfulness your efforts don't go unnoticed.

If we women do most of the food shopping and cooking, then we are the nutritional gate keepers. We are also equally the gate keepers for emotional support, comic relief, and all that is good in a relationship. Helping someone see that the choices they make can have enormous consequences on their health and wellness is the best gift we can give.

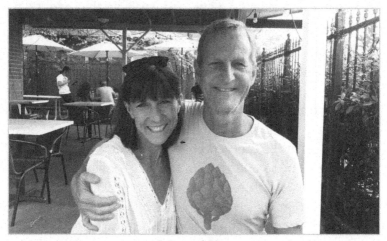

Me and He

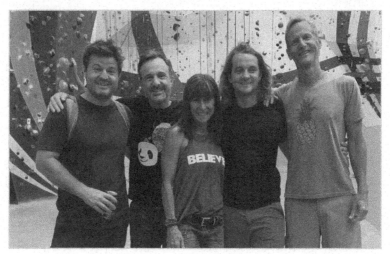

Us

TAKEAWAY TIPS

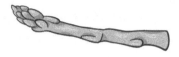

Plants, Purpose, and Partnership

These are my threesome of choice. Fuel you and your loved one well with purpose and passion and the power of plants, and I assure you that you will be blown away with what transpires.

Try for one week to:

- Eat a whole-food, plant-based diet, and take note of how you feel emotionally and physically.
- Define and then dive into a purpose. Any purpose will do; just choose something you are passionate about and commit whole heartedly for one week.
- Carve out time to be present and available 100 percent to your partner. No TV, no computer, no cell phone, no distractions between you. Allow for that time to ground your bond.

PENIS TIP –
PENISES ARE DELICATE

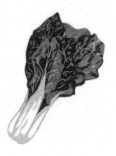

Penises and zippers do not belong in close proximity of each other. Why then is the zipper chosen to open and close pants? How about Velcro or snaps or even buttons? Nope. It has to be a line of sharp snarly teeth just waiting to close in on an unexpecting shaft. One of my least fond memories of early motherhood is zipping up my young son's penis. I would like to say this was a one and done occurrence—however, it was not. It was not my fault entirely as my sons were quite squirmy, and I was always in a hurry. I put "squirmy and hurry" in the same bucket as "zipper and pants." They don't go together. Oh, the horror of a penis caught in a zipper. To this day all three of my boys (men now) still have these unpleasant encounters etched in their memory banks of mom trying to untangle that mess. So sorry, boys.

Tip About the Tip

It is not just a zipper that can cause harm. Even though the male penis does not have a bone (unlike other mammals), the penis can still be broken. Not bone broken but blood-vessel broken—the blood vessels within the penis can burst and cause tremendous pain and swelling. And what are one-third of these cases attributed to according to the UK's National Health Service? — Sexual intercourse when you are on the bottom and your partner is on top. This is very brisk sexual intercourse, but I need to add none-the-less—ouch. And I bet if that partner was also using a zipper, the percentage would be higher.

ERECTILE DYSFUNCTION 101

Nothing will benefit human health and increase the chances for survival of life on Earth as much as the evolution to a vegetarian diet.

— Albert Einstein

If you are suffering from erectile dysfunction, you certainly don't need a 101. You are not a happy camper and neither probably is your sexual partner. You know very well what you are dealing with and how life altering it is. Before we dive into identifying what can be done to mitigate the issue at hand, let's look at the symptoms and reasons why erectile dysfunction (ED) is so prevalent among men of all ages. This is not just an older man's dilemma anymore. Just as we are seeing a rise in diabetes among children, we are also seeing ED in younger men.

One patient out of four with newly diagnosed erectile dysfunction is a young man. A man with a 42-inch waist is 50 percent more likely to have ED than one with a 32-inch waist. So guys, let's have a reality check. When naked, stand up straight and look down. Can you see your penis? It doesn't count if it is erect. You want to be able to see it in its limp state. If you can only see your belly, that is a problem. And if you can't see your penis perhaps your partner can't see it either.

Erectile Dysfunction is defined as "the recurrent or persistent inability to attain or maintain an erection in order to have satisfactory sexual performance." Thirty million men in the US and one hundred million men worldwide have some form of ED, and this is considered a "powerful predictor" to having a stroke or heart attack down the road. Forty percent of men over 40 have ED, and those who do have a 50-fold increased incidence of coronary artery disease (CAD). More on this in the next chapter.

High cholesterol, obesity, diabetes, stress, and smoking can all be contributing factors to erectile dysfunction. However, perhaps the most overlooked determinant by most men and their doctors is what you eat every day and how a poor diet can be the catalyst to the ailments listed above. This is the focus of this book. There is a clear correlation between ED and food. Eating foods that restrict blood flow is a huge part of the ED problem. If you know the facts about the origin of the issue and are armed with the right tools to not just mask the symptoms but actually attack the root cause, you have more control than you think you do. Let's look at the low-lying fruit so that your fruit flourishes.

An erect penis holds approximately eight times more blood than a flaccid one. In order to obtain and then keep an erection, the arteries into the penis fill with blood while the veins that transfer the blood back to the body close. The blood then is trapped thus granting the perfect erection. In a perfect world, the veins stay closed until after orgasm. The more trapped blood the better, and this leads to a firmer erection.

Constricted blood flow to the groin can lead to shorter-in-duration erections to nonexistent erections. This, I don't need to tell you, doesn't lead to being anywhere satisfying. Covered in detail in "The Canary in the Coal Mine" chapter, it explains that inadequate blood flow to the groin in many cases may be a danger sign to inadequate blood flow to the heart and to the brain. This can be a warning sign of things to come. Not enough blood flow to the groin is a sign that there is not enough blood flow throughout the body.

Let's talk about "endothelium." In the article written by cardiologist, Dr. Joel Kahn, MD, "What Does Sex Have to Do with Nutrition?" he explains the intricate interplay between our endothelium and the health of our arteries.

The article states:

> The endothelium is the single layer of cells lining all the arteries of the body. When

healthy, the endothelial lining of arteries makes a miraculous gas called nitric oxide that causes arteries to expand or dilate and also helps them resist clotting and athero-sclerosis (hardening of the arteries).

Nitric oxide production is not only crucial for the endothelial lining of the arteries that flow to the penis, it affects blood pressure, athletic performance, heart and brain health, and overall health in general. And what foods potentiate nitric oxide production? Plant foods.

The article goes on to state:

The endothelium can be injured throughout the body by poor lifestyle habits, such as smoking and consumption of animal-based and processed foods. Poor sexual perform-ance may result from endothelial damage and may be recognized years before the same disease process causes a heart attack.

As is pointed out in Dr. Greger's video, *Survival of the Firmest: Erectile Dysfunction and Death,* "Since the arteries that fuel the penis are so much smaller than the arteries that fuel the heart, a cheese burger, fries, and a shake could clog those smaller arteries up more quickly. The sooner we understand the relationship between the foods that we eat and our artery health, the sooner we clear the pipes and enjoy the benefits."

I really wanted this book to be a pop-up book. Nature has given us fabulous flavorful phallic foods to help us flourish. Think of how much fun it would have been to have fruits and veggies popping up throughout the book. Although fruits and veggies won't be physically popping out of the pages, they will be metaphorically. Each chapter highlights the benefits of eating from nature and the miraculous health benefits that ensue.

Food derived from animals doesn't pop up at all. There are no animal foods created by nature that are in any way pop-up-able. And hot dogs and sausage don't count because they are not food. According to the World Health Organization, these food-like products actually are classified as class one carcinogens that could potentially cause cancer.

In the movie documentary, *Forks Over Knives,* those interviewed on the topic of plant-based eating and erectile function were able to "raise the flag" better after switching to a plant-based diet.

And in the movie, *The Game Changers,* three college athletes were "put to the test" to see if penis erection quality and capability would be altered by either eating a meat or plant-based meal. These young guys were fed a meat centered meal on eve one and then a plant centered meal on eve two. These brave young men were then monitored while they slept on the frequency, duration, and robustness of their erections. The plant-based meal won in every category by a long shot.

There is a stigma swirling around the need to eat meat. The idea that you aren't a real man unless you eat meat is an outdated message. Eat meat because you love it but not because of any nutritional benefits. The largest strongest animals in the world all get their protein, calcium, and essential nutrients from the plant kingdom, and have you ever taken a look at their penises? No Viagra needed for the giant ape.

The first observational study in the relationship between ED and diet was conducted over a ten-year period by researchers from Harvard Medical School. Between the years of 2000 and 2008, over 25,000 men rated their sexual function and completed food questionnaires. Taking into account other factors (smoking, diabetes, cardiovascular disease) the men who ate more fruit had a lower rate of ED. This was associated with an increase of flavonoids in the diet (flavones, anthocyanins, and flavanones) that are potent antioxidants. (Refer to "The Power of Plants" chapter to see which foods make the cut.)

Changing your diet is the best tool in your tool box to combat erectile dysfunction. Smoking, lack of exercise, being overweight, high cholesterol, and high blood pressure are also contributors. But think about it—changing what you eat from a harmful diet to a health-promoting diet will lead to lowering your weight, cholesterol, and blood pressure. You will have more energy so that exercising will be a joy and not a job. Your healthy behavior will encourage you to hang out with more like-minded people who don't smoke so you will give up smoking. You will join running, rock climbing, and surfing clubs, and your erections will be epic.

Okay, maybe not all that will happen, but I do know that Bruce feels better than he ever has in his entire life because of his diet. He has more energy, a better outlook on the day, optimal weight, and a ginormous woodie multiple times a day. I am sure many more woodies pop up throughout the night that I am not even aware of. All of this despite living with advanced prostate cancer.

Up until nine years ago Bruce and I were SAD (Standard American Diet) eaters. We thought that meat was essential at every meal so we would get enough protein. We thought that gold fish crackers were a food group. And that milk and dairy products must be consumed for strong bones. We know now that meat of all types contains saturated fats and, in many cases, excessive amounts of protein. We know now that goldfish crackers are not a food group and that dairy of all types are perfect... for baby cows, not for humans.

In the article, "Is Meat Killing Us?" the authors looked at numerous studies and concluded:

> Even though limitations exist in these studies (e.g., lack of large, long-term randomized controlled trials; large amount of heterogeneity), avoidance of red and processed meats and a diet rich in plant-based whole foods including fruits, vegetables, whole grains, nuts, and legumes is a sound, evidence-based recommendation.

TAKEAWAY TIPS

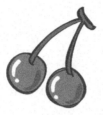

Erectile dysfunction can be caused by many factors that can be linked to a poor diet. Attack the root cause—improve the diet and see improvement from groin to heart to head. The connection between the foods we eat and our health outcomes are profound. So, with that in mind...

1. Be mindful about what you are choosing to eat and why. Eat animal products because you enjoy the taste, not for a powerful penis. The woodie needs blood flow and the foods that open the pipes are plants.

2. Join the following web sites and stay informed on all the current nutritional unbiased research and science and actionable items you can do to support your health. These are also found in the resource section.
    a. https://nutritionfacts.org/
    b. https://www.pcrm.org/
    c. https://nutritionstudies.org/
    d. http://www.foodrevolutionnetwork.org/
    e. https://aclm.memberclicks.net/

3. Watch Forks over Knives and The Game Changers movies! These powerful documentaries have triggered a global shift toward plant-based nutritional awareness.

PENIS TIP –
THE PENIS PUMP

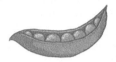

While Bruce was in recovery after his excruciatingly long robotic surgery to suck his prostate out of his belly button, the male nurse who was taking care of Bruce and I had a frank discussion. We didn't yet know the extent to which the cancer had spread or how invasive it was to his prostate. All I cared about was my husband's sexual function. It didn't even occur to me that the cancer had spread outside the prostate bed and we had bigger problems to come. The oncologist had assured me that the cancer was contained and that this surgery would eliminate the C word and we would be good as new. The doc did mention, however, that Bruce's sexual function might be compromised, so that was the only thing on my mind. Boy, would that focus change in just a few short days.

So here I am discussing penises with this nurse and he opens up to me that he has a penal implant that allows him to basically inflate or deflate his penis as needed. "Oh, really," I reply. I am really wanting to ask to see it—please oh pretty please, but I hold back. I feel hope flushing through my body. Bruce can surgically have a pump implanted, and we can have sex whenever we want. WHAT was I thinking? Not much, it appears at the time. I just wanted my husband in working order, that's all.

Tip About the Tip

Penal implants date back to the 16th century. Early penal implants included taking a part of a rib, or a whole one, and inserting it into the penis. That proved to be problematic. Well, I could have told them that. In the 1970s, a high-grade silicone rubber was created by the National Aeronautics and Space Administration (NASA). Apparently astronauts needed assistance too. This material was used to create the first penal implant. The inflatable penile prosthesis (IPP) was first introduced in 1973.

I am not at all judging anyone for going the route of penal pumps or implants. Heck, I contemplated it as well. Just consider your diet and incorporating plants. Plants are nature's perfect penis pump. Even when you least expect it, that pump is working away providing just the right blood flow for any occasion without having to inflate a thing. Just chew and swallow. I am not saying that you don't have to work at it mentally and physically. Just before doing anything as drastic as having something surgically implanted into your body, try changing your diet. Give it a shot and see what greater blood flow brings to your groin.

THE CANARY IN THE COAL MINE

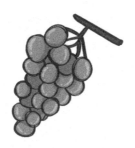

The beef industry has contributed to more American deaths than all the wars of this century, all-natural disasters, and all auto-mobile accidents combined. If beef is your idea of "real food for real people" you'd better live real close to a real good hospital.

— Neal D. Barnard

ED stands for early death.

— Dr. Michael Greger

Having ED may be a sign of health concerns much more serious. On NutritionFacts.org's website in Michael Greger's video, *Survival of the Firmest— Erectile Dysfunction and Death,* he summarizes numerous studies noting the plausible link between erectile dysfunction and coronary artery disease.

Coronary artery disease (CAD) "is the most common type of heart disease. It is the leading cause of death in the United States in both men and women. CAD happens when the arteries that supply blood to heart muscle become hardened and narrowed. This can lead to chest pain (angina) or a heart attack."

According to a newly published Physicians Committee for Responsible Medicine news release dated February 10, 2020, "A recent meta-analysis found that men with ED have a 59 percent higher risk of coronary heart disease or atherosclerosis, a 34 percent higher risk of stroke, and a 33 percent higher risk of dying from any cause, compared with men without symptoms of ED."

Erectile dysfunction symptoms show up before coronary artery disease. The penile arteries are approximately half the size of the coronary arteries and the same amount of plaque buildup would first clog the penal arteries limiting the amount of blood flow entering the penis. This is why so many men with signs of a heart attack had been living with ED for many years prior. It just takes longer for the coronary arteries to show the same signs. Penal clogged arteries are referred to as penal angina as "atherosclerosis is a systematic disorder that uniformly affects all major vascular beds"

(Michael Greger video, *Survival of the Firmest—Erectile Dysfunction and Death*). As Dr. Greger puts it, "ED stands for early death."

In Harvard Medical School's Special Health Report 2016 entitled "Erectile Dysfunction," Harvard's Dr. Michael P. O'Leary, the medical editor of the report, says that erections "serve as a barometer for overall health," and that erectile dysfunction can be an early warning sign of trouble in the heart or elsewhere.

In the "Erectile Dysfunction and Heart Disease" Cleveland Clinic article, it states "There is a very strong link between erectile dysfunction and heart disease. Several studies have shown that if a man has ED, he has a greater risk of having heart disease. In fact, having ED is as much a risk factor for heart disease as a history of smoking or a family history of coronary artery disease

Understanding that erectile dysfunction can be linked to an early death provides another reason for wanting to do everything you can to assure not only great sex but great health overall. As you read through this book and hopefully start applying what you have learned, remind yourself that what is good for the heart and head are good for the groin. It is that simple.

TAKEAWAY TIPS

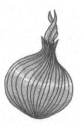

The human body has an amazing warning system put into place to alert us to any foul play afoot from top to bottom. As every action in our bodies has a reaction somewhere else in our bodies, it is no surprise that erectile dysfunction is a red flag for other more serious issues cooking up the vein chain. With this in mind, we need to take ED seriously—not only for the immediate sexual stuff, but for the more pressing—perhaps dropping dead of a heart attack stuff.

1. Erectile dysfunction is your body's alert system telling you that serious life-threatening, artery-clogging issues are happening in your body. Take heed and take action now.

2. Take control of your health now. Don't rely on a pill or a potion to reverse the effects of a poor diet. We all have more control over our health and happiness then we give ourselves credit for. There is no one in charge of your health but you.

3. When we were born, we were not automatically given a ticket to good health no matter what. We

weren't also given any road map, so we do the best we can with the information that we collect day to day. Unfortunately, many of us have been given the wrong guidance about the foods we should be eating to keep us healthy. It isn't our fault. However, it does become our fault entirely if we don't take action. If you know of someone with ED, the time is now for that person to take this seriously and opt for the best choices for a long healthy—and not compromised life.

PENIS TIP –
THE LITTLE BLUE PILL

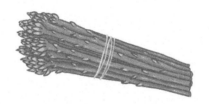

Want to have sex? Just pop a pill. This is a route to go and many men go this route, but there are some nasty side effects. When Bruce came out of surgery after having his prostate sucked out of his belly button by robots, the doctor gave us guidelines of how to get Bruce's erections back up and running, and one of those was to include a daily dose of Viagra whether or not sex was in the cards. We listened to the doc, and Bruce popped his pill every day—in the beginning. This seemed to work okay. However, there were the after effects. Bruce would turn a flush beet red, and he would feel like his head was going to explode and not in the wow orgasm way, but in the "holy crap my head is going to explode" way. And not the head you may be thinking.

Other than that, it was fine.... Hah! Sex with those side effects—no thank you. There had to be a better option. Luckily the more we adopted a whole food, plant-based diet and then with the no oil kicker (that is what took it down the finish line, outlined all later in the book), the need for that little blue pill was no more.

If you want to endure the side effects of external artificial blood flow agents that you ingest with a multitude of not-so-sexy aftershocks, then the suggestions in this book may not be for you, but one tenet Bruce and I always remind everyone who takes our One Day to Wellness program is "What's the downside?" What is the downside to giving a change in diet a chance? There isn't any. Giving foods a try to enhance blood flow and clear arteries instead of clogging them add only to an upside. There is no downside to giving this route a try. Getting an erection naturally and it staying around on its own until it's not needed anymore at any age is a pretty wonderful thing.

Tip About the Tip

Originally developed in 1989 as "UK-92480" by Pfizer-Viagra, the little blue pill, was designed to treat high blood pressure and angina, a chest pain caused by reduced blood flow to the heart.

The test subjects were responding differently to the drug then researchers expected. They noticed a strange side effect to the men after they took the drug. Penal perkiness. Well what is a drug manufacturer to do? Change course and quick. Rebrand, repackage, and repurpose—and Viagra was born.

THE POWER OF PLANTS

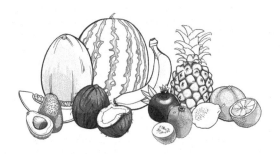

A human body in no way resembles those that were born for ravenousness; it hath no hawk's bill, no sharp talon, no roughness of teeth, no such strength of stomach or heat of digestion, as can be sufficient to convert or alter such heavy and fleshy fare.

— Plutarch

It's the Food

This chapter highlights the foods that create greater blood flow and generate more upward mobility to the groin area as well as improving overall health in general. As the old saying goes, "What's good for the goose is good for the gander." What fuels a healthy body overall is also what fuels a healthy hearty erection.

What are these magic sexual super foods? Before listing specific foods that enhance and promote everything below the belt, let's look at the big picture. There are those who may assume that a supplement will cure a nutrient deficient diet. There are others who exercise so that they can eat whatever they want thinking that the exercise alone will outweigh the over consumption of eating the wrong types of food. Some even presume there are super foods that, if eaten in isolation, will make up for all the other garbage that gets transported from mouth to stomach.

We have never been able to or never will be able to supplement our way to good health, or for that matter, exercise our way out of a bad diet. Super foods alone aren't enough if the overall landscape is poor. It is like planting one flower in a bed of weeds or cleaning out just one room in your house while leaving the other rooms filthy. Look at ALL that is contributing to the story. There is a balance and connection to the choices we make. Let's clean house and get rid of the weeds in the yard and fill our plate with super sexy foods that will help us flourish in all that is wellness. Below I have listed my favorites and ideas on how to easily add these foods into your daily lineup. You will also see many of these miraculous foods included in the recipes section.

Multiple studies point to the foods that adversely or positively affect our sexual functioning. As referenced earlier, findings from the Men's Professional Follow-up Study that followed over 25,000 men for over 10 years showed erectile improvement in the men who ate more plant foods, foods rich in antioxidants and flavonoids—phytonutrients found only in plants. "The more fruits and veggies in the diet, the better," the study cited. "Men who regularly consumed foods high in these flavonoids were ten percent less likely to suffer erectile dysfunction. In terms of quantities, we're talking just a few portions a week," stated lead researcher Aedin Cassidy, PhD. Dr. Cassidy's group wrote, "Our data strengthens the knowledge that a healthy diet, specifically one rich in several flavonoids together with increased physical activity and maintenance of body weight, are important components of health to improve sexual health and CVD risk factor reduction." The study noted that the men who ate the highest fruit flavonoids had a 14 percent reduction in ED risk.

Plant foods are rich in nitric oxide promoters, includeing nitrates, folates, and flavonoids. Nitrates are called vasodilators. Vasodilators open up blood vessels and increase blood flow. And as mentioned, it is all about the blood flow. The more nitric oxide promoting foods the better.

Nitrates / Nitric Oxide (NO)—Plant based nitrates, found in all dark leafy green vegetables, are metabolized and converted to nitric oxide that is delivered to our arteries and veins via the endothelial lining. A diet high in dark leafy greens provides the raw ingredients to one of the most powerful substances in the human body. For a nitric oxide shot, try beets or beet juice, leafy greens such as kale, arugula, spinach, and citrus fruit for their nitrate punch.

Folate / Folic Acid—Folate and magnesium are also blood-flow boosters as well as increasing testosterone levels. A deficiency of folic acid has been linked to erectile dysfunction.

Flavonoids

Flavonoids are phytonutrients (plant chemicals) that are found in almost all fruits and vegetables. Flavonoids, carotenoids, and flavons are antioxidants that help lower blood pressure and decrease cholesterol which can contribute to erectile dysfunction. Along with carotenoids that are responsible for the red, yellow, and orange pigments in fruits and veggies, flavonoids are also the reason for the bright colors in fruits and vegetables. From *Today's Geriatric Medicine,* (Vol. 6, No. 4, Pg. 30):

> Flavonoids are a subclass of polyphenols, "those plentiful and super-heart-healthy plant chemicals found in fruits and vegetables," says Janet Bond Brill, PhD, RDN, LDN, CSSD, a cardiovascular nutritionist and author of *Prevent a Second Heart Attack: 8 Foods, 8 Weeks to Reverse Heart Disease.* "In fact, they are the largest and most diverse subgroup, with more than 5,000 disease-fighting phytochemicals identified."

Nitrate rich whole-food, plant-based foods include:

Beets, Beet Greens, and Beet Juice

Why—Beets contain folate, vitamin C, fiber, and nitrates that have been shown to increase athletic performance and lower blood pressure. Studies show that drinking just 17 ounces of beet juice up to two-three hours before working out can increase athletic performance up to 25 percent.

How—Add beets and beet greens to smoothies or chopped up in salads. Don't throw the greens away. Instead cook them in a soup or stew. Drink a shot of beet juice before any athletic endeavor to see your performance improve.

Garlic and Onions

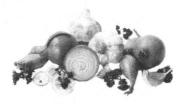

Why—Garlic and onions are part of the allium family which possesses the phytochemical allicin that helps thin the blood and aids in circulation. Garlic can make nitric oxide more bioavailable.

Just a word of advice—Eat these with your significant other as you won't notice the smell. Bruce and I eat garlic and onion almost at every meal and we smell so good—to each other. And this is all that matters. But if you aim to impress with your breath, chew on a little mint or parsley after your garlic party.

How—Add to any soup, stew, or stir fry. Try fresh, powered, raw, or cooked. Purchase dried chopped onion and garlic and sprinkle on literally anything. Check out Bruce's Killer Salad Dressing or my through-the-roof Oil-Free Hummus or Oil Free/Cheese Free Pesto in the recipes section.

Leafy Greens—arugula, kale, spinach, watercress, collards, cabbage, bok choy, Swiss chard.

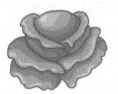

Why—Leafy green vegetables are packed with nitrates that then are converted to nitric oxide and as mentioned above nitric oxide opens up blood vessels and increases blood flow.

How—Fresh is best but frozen is fine and when in a pinch, canned without added salt is a shortcut. Basically, get your leafy greens in any way you can. Add to smoothies for breakfast, salads, and soups for lunch, stir fry at dinner.

Check out the wilted green recipe for breakfast. You can eat twice as many cooked greens as raw ones, and when wilting (just steaming your greens until they have "wilted" but not cooked to mush), you are not losing any of their nutritional benefits.

Watermelon

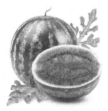

Why—We will highlight the watermelon rind in our stand outs super foods section but for right now eat the rind as well as the flesh—trust me.

How—Watermelon juice, watermelon by itself, watermelon in a salad. Buy an entire watermelon. Cut it up. Eat a ton and refrigerate or freeze the rest. The rind included.

Pomegranates

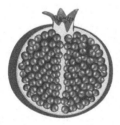

Why—Pomegranates have antioxidants that mitigate cell damage that helps protect the production of nitric oxide. One study showed that pomegranate juice was linked to improvement in reduction of artery plaque that can lead to endothelial dysfunction.

How—For a fast and easy ingenious way to get the seeds out of the pomegranate, check out our recipes section on our website, onedaytowellness.org. Bruce tackles the pomegranate underwater (no, he is not underwater—only the pomegranate) so that the seeds sink to the bottom of the bowl and the pulp rises to the top. He buys a case at a time, does the deseeding, and then he freezes the seeds and has them readily available to put into smoothies, on groats, salads, or just to eat alone as a great quick sweet snack.

Citrus Fruits—lemons, limes, oranges, grapefruit

Why—Citrus fruits, through their high vitamin C content, can potentiate the bioavailability of nitric oxide. Adding citrus fruit to other foods also enhances vitamin C absorption.

How—Blend; don't juice. Eat the whole fruit or include the entire fruit in a smoothie. Juicing citrus fruit removes all the fiber, and you are left with concentrated juice. The fiber is a crucial component to this flavorful package. This is how you should look at all fruit. In most cases, eat the whole package. This is what nature has provided to us. Where does much of the nutrition come from? The skin. Buy organic and eat the skin. Check out (in the recipes section) Bruce's lemon rind, turmeric, ginger snack if you want a nutritional power packed punch.

Nuts and Seeds—walnuts, cashews, peanuts, pine nuts, chestnuts, almonds, flax seed, chia seeds, hemp seeds

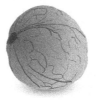

Why—Why not? Nuts and seeds are delicious, filling, and have just the right amount of healthy dietary-fat naturally found in the whole food. Nuts and seeds have an amino acid, arginine, that helps with nitric oxide production.

How—Play with your nuts and seeds, and pick the ones you like the best. My favorites—walnuts, pistachios, cashews, almonds, flaxseeds, chia seeds, hemp seeds, pine nuts. Pistachios get a special mention later on in the stand outs section.

Check out my amazing nut recipes—cashew cheese, cacao balls, pesto, even making your own nut butter is included. So easy and saves so much money.

Eat nuts for a snack or added to a recipe. Here is the tip about buying nuts—raw nuts are best, then dry roasted.

Steer clear of roasted nuts as that means most likely they were cooked with added oil.

A cautionary note about nuts though. If you are trying to lose weight or are trying to adhere to a lower fat diet, perhaps limit, but don't eliminate, your nut consumption.

A note about flax seeds. Eat one tablespoon every day. You will see this tip later on as well as this is an important addition to your diet. Grind them about every three days (we use a coffee grinder) and keep them either in the fridge or freezer as they oxidize quickly after being ground. But you want to eat them ground instead of whole as whole flax seeds go right through you without providing you with their nutritional gifts of antioxidants, protein, fiber, and alpha linolenic acid (ALA) which is a type of Omega 3 amino acid found in certain plant foods.

Dark Chocolate

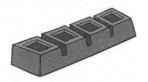

Why—Again, why not? Who doesn't love the cocoa bean? Cocoa contains antioxidants in the form of flavanols which promote increased nitric oxide levels.

How—All I can say is Hallelujah! Look for 72 percent and above. The darker the better. Check out my chocolate pudding recipe. Dip one of my cacao balls into the pudding for an added wow. Is chocolate better than sex or does having a piece of chocolate lead to having sex or lead to having better sex? Which came first—the sex or the chocolate? You be the judge. My recommendation—how about this sweet treat as the post glow goodie?

Folate-Rich Whole Food, Plant-Based Foods include:

Legumes—beans, peas, lentils

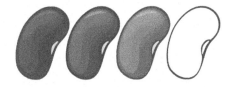

Why—One of the key tenets from the Blue Zones ("Blue Zone" is identified as geographic regions around the world where some of the world's oldest people reside) research by Dan Buettner and the National Geographic Society was that the longest-lived people in these "Blue Zones" primarily eat a whole-food plant-based diet includeing some sort of bean, lentil, or pea as a staple. In these communities where people are living measurably longer lives than the rest of the world, they all eat beans. Legumes are rich in fiber, protein, antioxidants, and folate.

How—This includes soy in the form of minimally processed organic soy. More about soy in the "Stand Outs and What Abouts" chapter. Include hummus on your morning toast, a taco bar at lunch, and bean stew for dinner.

And a special note to the black-eyed pea and the lentils for coming in at 358 mcg folate per cup.

Let's discuss the elephant in the room—flatulence. First off, farting is natural, and farting is fine. The sign of a healthy relationship is actually when you can fart in front of your partner. This is my personal opinion, and I stick by it. Have you ever gone on a date and needed to pass gas (just a small toot) and you didn't because you were too self-conscious? What a pent-up mess of a horrible date that was. I remember oh so well way back in the days when I was dating that all I wanted to do was to go home so I could relieve myself. Thankfully, I met my husband early in my life (I had just turned 21), and farting was fine between us. Bruce even taught our boys how to "cupcake." Okay, this is another thing that boys do that I totally don't get and also don't approve of in the least little bit. If you are unfamiliar about "cup caking," it's when you fart into your cupped hand and then proceed to cup your hand over the nose of whoever you happen to be with so that they can enjoy the full experience of the smell all to themselves. This is gross, but I guess that too is also a sign that the relationship is sound—I guess.

Anyway, let me get back to beans—farting may be an issue if you are adding legumes to a diet that currently is void of them. Start slow adding in one small serving and then more as your gut biome adjusts. On our video *Bean Basics* on onedaytowellness.org, we show you how to soak (overnight) then cook adding the spice, Epazote, found in many Mexican grocery stores or available on Amazon. More on this in our recipes section.

Epazote—this magical spice (leaf) is touted (not tooted) for its ability to reduce flatulence. Bruce and I swear by Epazote. And living closely in a 32-foot RV, we need all the gas reduction help we can find. And Bruce knows never ever is "cup caking" okay in the RV.

Cruciferous Vegetables—Brussels sprouts, cauliflower, kale, arugula, broccoli cabbage, bok choy, arugula, collards, watercress and radishes

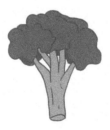

Broccoli

Why—Cruciferous vegetables are known for their high antioxidant, folate, fiber, vitamin, and mineral content

How—Roast Brussels sprouts or cauliflower cut in half on parchment paper in oven with balsamic vinegar, onion, and garlic powder. No oil needed. Steam broccoli, cabbage, and bok choy, and top with nutritional yeast for a cheesy flavor without the artery clogging cheese. Top avocado toast with arugula, watercress, and radishes.

Papayas and Mangos

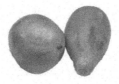

Why—These delicious tropical fruits are thought to possess aphrodisiac powers They are loaded with antioxidants, fiber, folate, and a number of studies show that regular consumption of mango helps to increase sperm count and reduce constipation. And let's be honest, constipation and sex don't mix in any setting.

How—papayas and mangos are so tasty and can be eaten alone or in smoothies or on top of salads. Fresh or frozen is fine.

Bananas

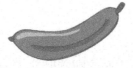

Why—Just look at a banana and tell me what that fruit is good for? They are thought to also be an aphrodisiac. Bananas aid in reducing constipation, assist with blood flow, and erection quality. Bananas are also thought to have a lot of potassium which they do, but here's an interesting fact—there are many other foods scoring higher on the potassium list. Compared to banana's, avocados, sweet potatoes, spinach, watermelon, coconut water, white beans, black beans, edamame, tomato paste, butternut squash, potatoes, dried apricots, Swiss chard, beets, and pomegranates all score higher.

How—How do you feel about ice cream? If ice cream is something on your "there is no way I can ever give it up" list, then I have the best healthier version alternative. Buy about-to-be-rotten bananas. Peel them and freeze. While you are waiting for the bananas to become frozen, purchase a YONANA ice cream maker.

This is THE gift I give for any and all occasions. The YONANA machine takes frozen, old, almost-rotten bananas and turns them into the best soft served ice cream you have ever tasted. Add any additional frozen fruit, cacao powder, nut butter, and you won't ever go back to health-harming dairy ice cream again.

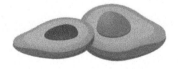

Avocado

Why—Interesting fact: Aztecs called the avocado tree the testicle tree. Besides being totally delicious, avocados are packed with healthy fat, fiber, and contain zinc that has been shown to increase testosterone levels.

How—I discuss oils in detail in the "Stand Outs and What Abouts" chapter. Use the whole food, and not its isolated oil. Avocado, as mentioned above, is loaded with fiber. That is the intact avocado. Not the oil that is pressed out of the avocado. Add avocado to pudding and brownie recipes. Top salads and soups and mash into avocado toast with lemon and pepper. There are many recipes incorporating avocados in the recipe section

Whole Grains

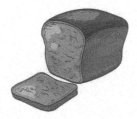

Why—Whole Grains have been shown to lower rates of ED because of their fiber, vitamins, and minerals that are linked to a healthy heart. The key is Whole Grain. I highlight this in more detail in my "Tips to Transition to a Healthier You."

How—Look for bread made from 100% whole grain including wheat, barley, spelt, einkorn, or rye. Make sure to read the label as enriched flour is not whole grain. As you will see in all my recipes, I only use whole grain. Eat whole grain groats (the whole intact grain) for breakfast.

Use whole grain rye bread for your hummus sandwich at lunch. Choose whole wheat pasta for your spaghetti at dinner.

Also, on the folate list are beets, citrus fruits, leafy greens, nuts, and seeds as mentioned above.

Special note to spinach on my Stand Out List—for topping out at 263 mcg folate per cooked cup.

Flavonoid Rich Whole Food, Plant-Based Foods

Berries and colorful fruits including blueberries, black berries, cherries, and black currents—but don't limit yourself to just these. Look for fruits with dark, deep color.

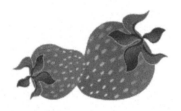

Why—These colorful fruits are also packed with anthocyanins, powerful antioxidants that protect artery function—the colors are the antioxidants so eat the rainbow of colors coming naturally from fruits, not Fruit Loops.

How—Eat berries and fruit on toast, pancakes, or oatmeal for breakfast. Have a fruit salad for lunch. Fruit is great for pies and muffins. Snack on fruit instead of fruit-flavored processed junk. Again—Fruit Loops are not fruit.

Indian Spices

We love to use different kinds of spices for all of our cooking and baking, and Indian spices including saffron, fenugreek seeds, cardamom, clove, fennel, ginseng, nutmeg, and ginger.

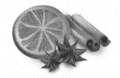

Why—These spices have the ability to enhance the flavor of food. Think of them as super-charged anti-oxidants. Many of these spices are also touted for their natural energy boosters and aphrodisiac enhancers. For example: Hot Pepper—in one study, men who spiced their food with pepper sauce had higher testosterone levels.

How—Play with these spices wherever you see fit. Bruce and I go crazy with these in stir fries, soups, and stews. For my baked goods, I love using nutmeg, ginger, cardamom, and clove. Don't be afraid to experiment. You never know how good a cook you can be unless you play with spices

TAKEAWAY TIPS

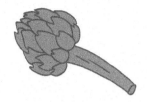

Food is powerful medicine capable of health promotion and extension. Specifically, for erectile function and blood flow to the entire artery and vein chain, eat foods high in nitrates, folates, and antioxidant flavonoids.

1. Eat nitrate-rich foods for increased blood flow and circulation.
2. Eat folate-rich foods for increased blood flow and circulation.
3. Eat antioxidant-rich foods for increased blood flow and circulation.
4. Get it! It all boils down to BLOOD FLOW.

PENIS TIP –
NIGHTTIME AND EARLY A.M.
ERECTIONS

The wake up woodie actually has a name. It is called a morning glory. I am very familiar with the morning glory. Have I mentioned that Bruce and I live in a fruit and veggie wrapped RV that is only 32 feet in length? These 32 feet consist of a cab for driving, a living area which includes the kitchen, a small bathroom, and a very small bedroom. Every morning I wake up before Bruce, make coffee, and proceed to launch into work on my computer. About an hour in, I feel a rocking sensation coming from the bedroom. It starts getting faster and more turbulent. Ahhh—the Morning Glory! This is what happens many mornings on a plant-based diet for us. The plants have been doing their work all night, and Bruce has woken to a wild, wonderful woodie. Twenty-four seconds pass, and it is quiet again, and Bruce is asking for coffee.

Tip About the Tip.

On average, a healthy man has three to five erections during a full night's sleep, with each erection lasting 25 to 35 minutes.

No one really knows the cause of night-time erections. Some studies suggest that night-time erections are connected to periods of sleep called the rapid eye movement (REM) sleep. This is when dreaming is most likely to take place.

Whatever their cause, most doctors agree that night-time erections are a sign that everything is working as it should.

STAND OUTS AND WHAT ABOUTS?

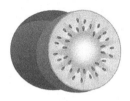

Let food be thy medicine, and medicine be thy food.

— Hippocrates

When diet is wrong, medicine is of no use.
When diet is correct, medicine is of no need.

— Ayurvedic proverb

There are some specific foods that have been studied that show promise for their potent erectile functioning attributes.

These are:

- Spinach
- Watermelon
- Pistachios
- Coffee

There are also foods worthy of accolades that have been given a bad-wrap by mostly rumor and innuendo—namely "soy" and those that have been given a pass when research doesn't warrant it—processed oil.

Wine is a hit or miss depending on the study cited so we will look at the best data to date. I wish consuming wine were more of a hit—we all love to hear good news about our bad habits. And being the wine lover that I am, I jump up and down clutching my glass of pinot when a study comes out touting the benefits of red wine. But the science points toward less than more, so even though I do drink wine, it is much less than I used to, and getting less and less. Damn you unbiased, not-for-profit research and science.

Then there are those foods that we hear are right on the money when it comes to sexual arousal and performance, but then again, we look to the cumulative research data available, and the conclusions are varied. Oysters and fish in general are in this category. We will discuss, and you then need to dive a little deeper into the science to see where you will dock your boat on this one.

Spinach

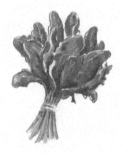

Spinach is packed with folic acid and a good source of magnesium which helps dilate blood vessels. One cup of cooked spinach contains 66 percent of RDA's folic acid requirement We were first introduced to the benefits of spinach in 1929 when the comic strip featuring Popeye the sailor man let us in on his secret weapon for building muscle. Popeye's biceps grew right after sucking down a can of spinach. Did you ever wonder what was going on below his belt as his biceps grew? Only Olive Oyl knows for sure.

In the same cartoon we were introduced to Popeye's pal, Wimpy. Wimpy is portrayed as sluggish, overweight, and not at all a sexual dynamo. All Wimpy eats are hamburgers. "I'll gladly pay you Tuesday for a hamburger today."

Popeye is slim and trim and full of energy. Popeye knows best, "I yam what I yam." "I am what I am, and that's all that I am." "I'm strong to the finish 'cause I eats me spinach."

Pistachio Nuts

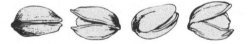

Pistachio nuts are a tremendous source of anti-oxidants, can contribute to lowering cholesterol, and have the amino acid arginine which is a known blood vessel relaxer. Studies show that men who eat more pistachio nuts have lower rates of ED, lower cholesterol levels, and have firmer erections.

Interesting note about pistachios also is that pistachios have protein, vitamin B6, and magnesium that can help you fall asleep. So instead of popping a melatonin pill to fall asleep, how about eating some pistachios?

Watermelon

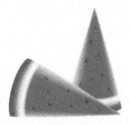

Watermelon leads the charge for L-circulene, an amino acid protein that converts to L-arginine that has the ability to relax blood vessels that lead to enhanced nitric oxide production and increased blood flow. This L—circulene is especially found in the watermelon rind. Yes, the rind you usually throw away. Watermelon has been thought to be an aphrodisiac. Dianne Hoppe, obstetrician, gynecologist, and author of *Healthy Sex Drive, Healthy You: What Your Libido Reveals About Your Life* states, "All that citrulline results in increased blood flow, blood vessel relaxation, and sexual arousal."

Coffee

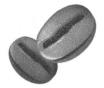

The caffeine in coffee boosts your metabolism, is loaded with antioxidants, and can affect blood flow. According to a study published in the journal *PLOS* in 2015 that included 3700 men, it was found that men drinking two-three cups of coffee lowered their ED risk by around 40 percent. Watch out though about drinking caffeine late in the day as it might interrupt your sleep.

In the Health Professionals Follow-Up Study, the research found a "strong inverse association between coffee consumption and risk of lethal prostate cancer."

Soy

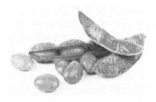

Let's talk about soy. For whatever reason soy—that sweet innocent little bean—has been demonized by the media, the barista at Starbucks, and perhaps even your doctor. Soy causes breast cancer. Soy grows boobs in boys. Soy is the worst food you can consume on the planet. You hear about the evils of soy, and after a while you just accept it as truth. This is not your fault. The more we hear about something—true or not—the more this message is instilled in us. It is how the rumor mill runs. The more we hear something about something, the more that something becomes truth.

Without going into excruciating detail on the benefits of soy—yes, you read that right—the benefits of soy. Let's just look at a population who eats a whole lotta soy, way more than us in the USA, the Japanese. If you look at their rates of hormonal cancers, the ones we would assume would be driven by our hormones—prostate and breast—and compare those rates to ours, their incidence of developing those cancers are orders of magnitude below ours. And yet they—the Japanese people—consume on an average, magnitudes more of soy than we do. There are many research studies citing the benefits of soy and perhaps limiting cancer incidence.

A super special mention to soy as soy consumption has been associated with a decreased risk of developing prostate cancer. Bruce and I add organic soy milk to our morning coffee. We top our salad at lunch with minimally processed organic tofu. At least once a week we make a stir fry with mushrooms and tempeh. And you have to try my chocolate pudding made with silken tofu. This recipe is to die for. Yes, you can put the book down now, run to the store to buy the ingredients, and make my pudding. Go now. Eat soy!

Red Wine

The same professionals' Follow-Up Study cited earlier led by Harvard University and the University of East Anglia did show that men who consumed more flavonoid rich foods had lower rates of ED, and this included red wine. Keep in mind that blueberries, strawberries, apples, pears, radishes, and citrus fruit are rich in flavonoids which are all antioxidant rich foods. On the flip side there are studies showing that no amount of alcohol is health promoting. And overconsumption is never a good idea—just saying this from personal experience, "The willie doesn't perform tipsy." Wine makes for a wilted woodie. I have also witnessed the willie to wander with too much wine, and as you will read later in the book, Bruce says NO cheating under any circumstances. So take heed, and if you choose to drink, keep it tidy.

The ISSUE with OIL

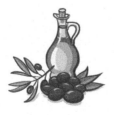

We have discussed the benefits of whole plant foods for erectile function. Let's now discuss one manufactured food product that is thought to be health promoting when, in fact, many studies show that the opposite is perhaps true, and this is oil. All oil—yes, even olive oil and coconut oil and avocado oil. All oil is 100% manufactured free fat. This means that the fat has been isolated from the food it was derived from. It has been separated from the nutrients and the fiber and the goodness of the whole plant food and sold to us as a magic elixir when in fact it is 100% liquid fat. Our bodies aren't meant to eat isolated fat. Fat is an essential macronutrient found in plants and we do need it, but nature never intended for us to adulterate the plant and extract the fat, leaving all the nutrition behind.

Studies have shown that consuming oil may "injure our arteries and promote heart disease because they increase inflammation." In the article "Olive Oil Nutrition—What's Wrong with Olive Oil? Separating the Truth from Hype," written by Senior Editor and Writer of the Pritikin Longevity center, Eugenia Killoran says,

> Hype: The Mediterranean diet is a heart-healthy diet, and it's rich in olive oil, so olive oil must be heart healthy and the key to a longer life.

> Truth: The people on earth with the longest life expectancy and the least heart disease do *not* eat diets rich in olive oil or any other fat. They *do* eat a diet rich in whole, natural foods like vegetables, fruits, whole grains, and beans.

When eating added fat, just remember:

1. All oil is 100% fat.
2. Oil is manmade and is a processed food.
3. Oil is void of almost all vitamins and nutrients.
4. There is no fiber in oil. All the fiber has been removed in the processing.
5. Oil is calorically dense coming in at 120 calories per tablespoon.
6. Eat fats naturally occurring in the food—not extracted from it.

So, what about oysters and other sea food?

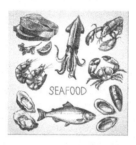

When you ask the question, you should add, "Compared to what?" There are some camps that say seafood is better than other meats. There are even research studies showing the benefits to eating fish. My cards say that there are better options—for our health and the health of the fish. Our oceans unfortunately have turned into the dumping grounds for mercury, dioxins, and other pollutants that harm the fish, and in turn, harm those who chose to eat the fish. Do your own research and determine the risks-toreward ratio. Bruce and I don't eat fish anymore. Fish was one of the last things to go off our plate. Do we miss it? Frankly, no. Because our plates are full of the bounty of nature's garden.

TAKEAWAY TIPS

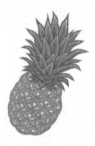

Although there are stand-out foods that have been tested individually for their ED potential, don't lose sight of an over-all health-promoting diet. Eating these stand-out foods will enhance a diet already rich in essential nutrients and antioxidants but not take the place of a healthy diet

1. Make your next salad be a watermelon, spinach, and pistachio salad.
2. If you drink coffee, keep at it two to three cups and not too close to shut eye. Also try green tea or maca for their high antioxidant capacity.
3. Give up oil for one week and see how you feel. And if you eat fish or oysters, eat them because you love them and not for the health benefits

PENIS TIP –
DON'T JUDGE A MAN'S PENIS SIZE BY THE SIZE OF HIS FEET

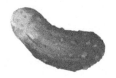

I grew up surrounded by penises. I had a dad, of course, and he helped make three young penises and me— the lone vagina in this sea of penises. My mom was a wonderful, opened minded, smart, gifted, savvy role model in every way except the way of the penis. She would protest in no uncertain terms that all penises were the same size when erect, so if you have seen one, well, you have seen them all. She was adamant that she was correct on this matter. This was coming from a woman who I think only had ever seen one erect penis. I also think this was her way of encouraging me to be monogamous to only one person and not to be curious as to what else was out there. I have been happily monogamous for close to 40 years, but sorry mom, before that, I saw my share of erect penises and I learned very quickly that mom's knowledge of the erect penis was limited to only one woodie.

Tip About the Tip

What I learned through my personal and then pro-fessional research was that mom wasn't at all correct. Men are either "showers" or "growers" meaning that, when flaccid, the size of the penis is all over the map. According to a 1996 article in the *Journal of Urology*, "There's no way to predict the size of a man's erect penis when it's flaccid. However, a stretched-out penis is a good predictor of its ultimate erect size." This is coming from a 2000 study in the *International Journal of Impotence.*

According to a 2013 study, the average penis size erect is 5.6 inches long. There are of course larger and smaller penises out there. The largest penis to date and recorded comes in at 13.5 inches when erect. Don't mean to call you out dude, but—"Go Johan Falcon."

It turns out that shorter penises when flaccid have larger erections. Research shows that shorter penis lengths when flaccid grow by 86 percent when erect as oppose to longer flaccid penises growing only 47 percent.

In the 1988 study published in the *Journal of Sex Research,* researchers also found that the difference in length between a short penis and a longer one was a lot less obvious when erect than when flaccid. For example, the flaccid penises varied in length by 3.1 cm (1.2 inches), whereas the average erect lengths differed by only 1.7 cm (0.67 inches).

Oh yes, and the foot myth. Well, it turns out that there is no correlation between foot size and penis size. The *International Journal of Impotence Research Trusted Source* published an Iranian study looking at other correlations. They concluded that "penile dimensions are significantly correlated with age, height, and index finger length," but not foot size.

TAKING MATTERS LITERALLY INTO YOUR OWN HANDS

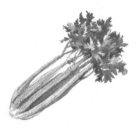

Some people think plant-based diet, whole-foods diet is extreme. Half a million people a year will have their chests opened up, and a vein taken from their leg and sewn onto their coronary artery. Some people would call that extreme.

— Caldwell Esselstyn

The future depends on what we do in the present.

— Gandhi

S orry about the title of this chapter—that one was just sitting there. Taking matters into your own hands refers to taking action NOW. You have read the great news about the power of plants, so it is time to eat them.

71

What is the downside? There isn't any. Only upside to your health and happiness. But behavioral change is hard. You have been told your entire life that animal products are good for you and you have to include them at every meal. This has been your plan, and now there is a new plan. A better plan, but where to start? Let's start where it matters—navigating your plate.

3G Strategy

High-fat animal and processed foods are shown to clog arteries and veins and restrict blood flow to not only the penis but to the heart and brain as expressed in the chapter, "Canary in the Coal Mine." Foods that drain our energy and that don't support our immune system or health in general should be low on our grocery list. This includes meat, dairy, and most processed foods.

Eating more fruits and veggies, whole grains, and beans and legumes crowds out the not-so-healthy foods that usually play a starring role on your plate. Learning to "Lean to the Green" as Bruce and I coin it is following our "3-G Eating Strategy" otherwise known as 3G. It is so simple and doesn't require calculators, counting calories, or counting macros. You just fill up your plate with plant foods first. These are greens and grains. Think ALL plant foods, including all fruit and vegetables, these are the Greens—then potatoes, beans, peas, lentils, whole grains - anything whole-food plant-based.

Then and only then if there is any room left on the plate, include, what we call the guilty pleasure. Maybe your guilty pleasure is a slab of some sort of meat. Maybe it is a cheese and pepperoni pizza. Or perhaps a mac and cheese with cheese on top. Choose your favorite and include it on your plate, but only put that food on the smallest sliver you have left as all the rest of your plate is covered with greens and grains. By consuming the healthiest food at the first course, you will be training your taste buds to actually prefer these foods and you will be full before even getting to your guilty pleasure so you will eat less of it. You won't feel deprived at all as the 3G Eating Strategy doesn't strip you of the foods you are used to eating. 3G just suggests you eat your guilty pleasure last after you have filled up on the good stuff.

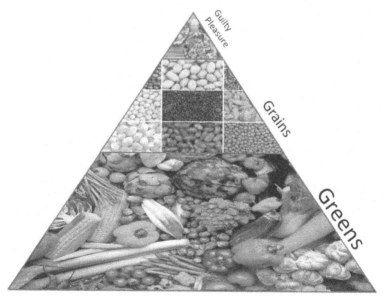

Let's get more specific about the 3G strategy.

Basically, 3G is turning the standard American diet on its head. Instead of meat and dairy being the star of the show, greens and grains are. Just flip the plate in reverse of what you may currently be doing and you've got it. Here is what the 3G Eating Strategy looks like.

G1—Greens. This course is mandatory. Greens is a blanket term for all veggies and fruits. Fill most of your plate or bowl with either fresh, raw, steamed, or sautéed (no oil), dark leafy green vegetables along with other colorful vegetables such as carrots, mushrooms, squash, tomatoes, onions. The more the better. Always eat this serving first or in combination with grains outlined in G2.

For breakfast, fresh berries (blue, black, raspberries) can take the place of greens. Berries are the most nutrient dense fruits, and because of all the natural fiber, they will not raise your blood sugar levels like refined sugar products. Include other fruit and veggies throughout the day as well as delicious snacks.

G2—Grains. This course is mandatory. Make sure to include a healthy portion of high-quality whole grains and starches with your meal. This course can be eaten either after G1 or in combination with G1. Beans, beans, beans—did I mention beans? White beans, black beans, chickpeas, edamame, and pulses (beans). Pulses (beans), as they are also referred to, are one of the most nutrient-dense foods in the plant kingdom that have also been shown to improve satiation when transitioning to a plant-based diet. These foods play a common theme among the longest-lived people from the Blue Zones research. They all eat some form of bean. Also include sweet potatoes, wild rice, brown rice, and groats. If you love white rice, just make sure you choose it less often as white rice has had many of its nutrients removed during processing. And there are many more nutritious options available.

For breakfast, steel cut oatmeal or unsweetened muesli with your fresh berries are an excellent choice—and fruit as a snack should always be your go-to.

G3—SIDE DISH or Condiment. This course is OPTIONAL and should be eaten last. This is your comfort food or guilty pleasure. Make sure it is a food that you love (if it's kale salad, you are in a good spot). Make it a big enough portion so that you feel you have deprivation insurance on your plate. If you can stick with this plan for six weeks, you will find that you begin losing your desire for the guilty pleasure. This guilty pleasure should be as small as possible but big enough so you don't feel deprived. Remember, it's a condiment on your plate that you are trying to reduce and or eliminate from your daily meals when you are ready. Take as much time as you need. Reduce your guilty pleasure at your own pace that you know you can sustain.

That's it! Simple, right? Too simple, you may say? The simpler something is the more adherence there is. Nature made eating simple. Humans were the ones to come along and make eating so complicated. This is one of the reasons why we are in the disease mess we are in today. Hold my hand, and I will help you navigate this new course. With just a small amount of guidance you will be the master of your domain.

Food Prep takes too much time - or does it?

Let's dissect a 24-hour day and see where we can squeeze in a little food prep time. Prepping is the key to always having available what you need when you need it. We eat nutritionally devoid food because it is cheap, easy to grab and go, and we think it is tasty because our taste buds have been hijacked by too salty, too sugary, too fatty, overly processed, fantasy food-like products that aren't really food at all.

Let's approach preparing and cooking as a gift we give to ourselves and to our loved ones. With a small amount of thinking ahead, we will never be stuck resorting to nutritionally depleted food-like products ever again.

Start the night before by soaking the A.M. groats—kamut, oat, farrow, buckwheat. These groats can also be used as the grain for lunch and dinner meals as well.

More about groats and beans (garbanzo, black, pinto, black-eyed peas) in the recipe section. Soak enough for three days. This will require two-three minutes total prep time. Rinse first the groats and or beans—then put them into a bowl with a ⅓ ratio of groats/beans to water. If you are having fresh fruit on your A.M. groats, you can cut these up and place them in an air-tight container in the fridge. With the chopping and the soaking done, you are in for around ten minutes.

On the first day of your new food prep routine, wake up one hour early. You will only need to do this on day one.

Day One: Drain the soaking water off both grains and beans and replace with new water around 1-2 ratio groats/beans to water. Cook both the groats and the beans—in separate pots, of course. The groats don't take very long. Depending on the groats you choose, check at ten minutes and then keep checking every five minutes after that until the groats reach the consistency that you like. You want them chewy and al dente and not mushy. My groats never take more than 15-20 minutes to cook. Put on a pot of coffee or tea and while you are waiting for the groats to get al dente, perform the following: 50 pushups, 50 squat jumps, 50 split lunges, and hold a plank for one minute. You have now done part of your workout routine for the day while cooking both breakfast and part of dinner (the beans). You are now 20 minutes in.

Serve the groats with one tablespoon of ground flax seed, a splash of unsweetened motherless milk (soy, almond, oat, hemp), fresh berries, banana, currents, and a handful of walnuts. You are 35 minutes in.

Check the beans. Depending on the bean, they are either done or need about 10-20 more minutes. Repeat the same total body strength workout. Drink a large glass of water and perhaps another round of coffee/tea. You are now close to 60 minutes in. Let's look at your invested 60 minutes

You have made and eaten the most nutritious breakfast on the planet and have enough left over for two more days. You have made beans that will go into a taco salad for dinner tonight, a stir fry tomorrow night, and a soup on eve three. You might even have enough left over to whip up some no-oil hummus for spreads of every type. You have completed a killer total body strength workout and all this in about an hour. By spending 10 minutes last night and one hour this A.M., you have saved time and money and gained health benefits from every angle.

Tomorrow A.M. you will not have to wake up early as everything was done today. However, you may just want to wake up early as today was so damn productive and an awesome way to start the day. When the day starts right, it usually stays right!

What I just outlined is not about finding one hour and ten minutes extra in your day. It is about changing your priorities. And changing priorities changes the trajectory of the rest of your life. What can be more important than to fuel yourself properly for the day ahead, to get the blood flow pumping early so you are ready for anything the day presents? This is your choice, and the rewards you reap from a small amount of preplanning are the game changer.

TAKEAWAY TIPS

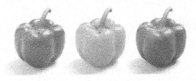

The 3G eating strategy is smart, sustainable, and satiating. A traditional diet either leaves you starving or feeling deprived. These diets don't work for the long haul and almost always fail. What 3G so brilliantly does is recalibrates your taste buds without restricting calories. You start craving the health-promoting foods and in turn push away the disease promoting foods.

1. Reverse your plate—Greens and Grains are the main event on your plate with your guilty pleasure saved for last. Make your guilty pleasure portion only enough for just a few bites. You don't need any more than one to three bites to be satisfied.
2. Make food prep an event that includes mindfulness and movement. You can get so much done in just one hour when you plan and prioritize.
3. Start thinking of food as part of you. Food is not something that you just eat. Food is a partnership. You treat it well with thoughtfulness and your time, and it will in return unleash a bounty of energy, vitality, and life.

PENIS TIP – THERE REALLY IS A PENIS MUSEUM

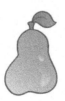

If you are wondering where to go for your next vacation, wonder no more. Iceland is where it's at for penis parts. It is there you will find the world's largest collection of penises in the world. An Icelandic history teacher named Sigurður Hjartarson, in 1974, was given a cattle whip made out of a bull penis as a gift. This sparked the notion in his brain that surely there could be other penises to collect and the Icelandic Phallological Museum was born. The museum holds a collection of more than 238 penises and penile parts.

The largest penis at the museum comes from that of a sperm whale. It's six feet tall and weighs just shy of 150 pounds. I am so glad I am not a female sperm whale. Imagine seeing that thing coming at you. Just saying. "You'll learn that as with everything in nature, the diversity in this department is as great as in any other; even within the same species the difference in size and shape is often quite remarkable," Hjartarson told Mental Floss in 2015.

TANGIBLE TRANSITIONING TIPS

First, nutrition is the master key to human health. Second, what most of us think of as proper nutrition—isn't.

— T. Colin Campbell

One farmer says to me, "You cannot live on vegetable food solely, for it furnishes nothing to make the bones with": and so he religiously devotes a part of his day to supplying himself with the raw material of bones; walking all the while he talks behind his oxen, which, with vegetable-made bones, jerk him and his lumbering plow along in spite of every obstacle.

— Henry David Thoreau

The frame work is 3G—Greens, Grains, and Guilty pleasure. Eat more fruits and vegetables, whole grains, and beans. Cut out processed food and eliminate or drastically reduce your intake of anything animal based in order to live a life full of fun and frolic. But HOW? Like most people who learn the WHY, the HOW is the most difficult to tackle as the How is about changing behavior. The How is actually taking action. Think of all the things you know you should do but haven't implemented even with best intentions. This is not your fault. Look around you at all the obstacles in your way. You have pressure to stay the same from every vantage point. Switching what you eat is huge and could potentially shift the game in so many ways. Dan Buettner author of the *Blue Zones* offers this piece of advice to doctors to advise their patients, "Make friends with people who eat a whole-food plant-based diet because healthy behaviors are contagious."

You may find your friends don't like at all that you are choosing healthier behaviors. You might be down-right shunned, but stick with it, and as you start to notice a healthier you, so will they, and they will want to know your secret. Anyone can follow the current status quo, but it takes a leader to lead. Health, wellness, and woodies sell, and you will be the perfect salesperson. If Bruce, my carnivore sceptic husband, could make this transition, you can too. Below are simple tangible tips for transitioning to a leaning to the green, incorporating the 3Gs, and living a Whole-Food Plant-Based life.

These tips and tricks are tried and true and ready for you to implement into your life today. It is the way in which you design your steps that is key to your success. In order to change behavior, you need to distinguish yourself as either a dipper or a diver. You may be both depending on the circumstance.

The Dipper

A dipper is someone who changes his or her behavior by taking small steps. One step that sticks will then lead to the next step, and before you know it, you are making your way down the path to creating sustained change. An example of this might be the following.

> Meat has saturated fat that can clog your arteries and veins and may lead to limited blood flow that can cause erectile dysfunction. You love meat. There is no way you are going cold turkey. You love turkey. And if you were to try to dive in and make changes too quickly, you would just fail and that would lead to not wanting to take the next step. The first dip should be something that you know you can do. Something small that will be easy for you to stick with and win with. That WIN will provide the satisfaction you need to dip again.

> So if you love meat and eat some form of meat product at every meal, how about

83

trying just one meal a day to be meat free? (I have outlined very simple recipe ideas in the recipe section and also in the shortcuts section for you to try.) This may look like instead of eggs for breakfast choose a tofu scramble. Or instead of a smoked turkey sandwich at lunch, choose a hummus and veggie sandwich. For dinner, choose a veggie pizza instead of pepperoni pizza. As a dipper, change one meal and see how that goes then continue to make small changes as you see success.

The only downside to dipping is that with small changes come small results. You may not see a huge difference right away and might get frustrated—literally. Know this going in—that you are walking the marathon and not running it. You will get there. It will just take a little longer.

The Diver

Now a diver is someone who has experienced the WHY and can't look back. Knowing the WHY is enough to take and make drastic changes right away. Bruce and I are divers. Once we know we can't "unknow" the information. It is like being locked in a bad unhealthy space and you so badly want to get out. You locate the key to unlock the door, and you get out of that space. You don't put the key in your pocket and just hang out in that unhealthy space. This analogy is what I call my mind shift. I know, and I can't "unknow," so what am I going to do about it? I am going to take action right away. Creating this mind shift has allowed me to construct the following tips for you. It is easier than you think when your focus is on health, well-being, and the long game—literally. This means a long game of amazing sexual experiences that leave you exhilarated and not deflated.

TIPS TO TRANSITION TO A HEALTHIER YOU

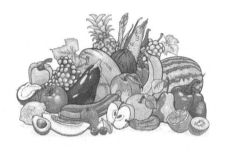

1. The Mind Shift

Trying to change our behavior takes time and effort. We may feel anxious thinking that we will be deprived of the comfort foods we have grown to love over the course of our lives. It's really tough. But the good news is that we now have more tools at our disposal based on years of solid scientific evidence and case studies of what actually DOES work in the long haul!

In October 2009 the Economic and Social Research Council, a British research group, released 129 different studies on behavioral change strategies. Bottom line: Most people attempt to implement self-behavioral change because of a sense of guilt, fear, and/or regret. And if your motivation to change is rooted in any of these feelings, your odds for achieving long term success are slim to none.

The same studies showed that creating just a few specific goals—"I'll eat a salad for lunch every day" instead of "I am going to try to eat healthier" consistently have the best results in the long haul. In addition to creating a few, simple goals, the analysis of the studies also indicates the vital importance of having a simple, specific road map to get you where you want to go. The more entrenched the habit, the harder it is to change. Obviously, some behaviors take much longer to alter than others. The most difficult behaviors to change—quitting smoking, quitting drinking, changing what you have learned and loved to eat your entire life—are a lifelong work in progress that requires attention every day for the rest of your life. The great news is that this new you that you are creating is thriving and is looking forward and not backward. And the old habits you tossed are not returning because you love the new you.

Remember, serious behavioral change is an ongoing process requiring fine tuning and changing tactics, not a one-time sprint to a finish line only to return to your old ways.

The five stages of behavior are easy to understand and make perfect sense. The KAIPA model below stresses the importance of understanding the REASONS behind your desire to change. From this knowledge base, you can now progress up the ladder of behavioral change to self-approval to make the change, creating intention to do so, actually implementing the practice, and finally advocating the change to others. This sequence of events more closely represents my journey to becoming a plant-based eater. First came the knowledge. At age 48, I read several books regarding the scientifically proven health benefits of plant-based eating. I quickly approved of this knowledge based on credibility of the authors and validation by research and science, and started up the path to practicing a total plant-based diet, to finally advocating it to others.

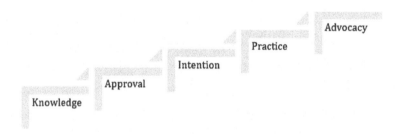

In the book *Atomic Habits* by James Clear, he outlines how our habits shape our identity. Focus on creating habits based on who you want to become—*identity based habits*—rather than choosing to change behavior for the short term to reach a short turn goal—*outcome-based habits*. The identity-based habits seem to stick whereas the outcome-based habits are fleeting. I want people to see me as someone whose habits represent my values and purpose and are part of who I am. Therefore, I do not choose to change habits by following the latest fads. This is a short-sightedness mindset that only leads to short-term success with failure lurking around the corner.

What do others say about you? Are you consistent? Focused? Purposeful? In order to change behavior, if that is your goal, you need to know the why and then pave your path forward with reinforcements for when the going gets tough. That all starts and continues with your mindset. When establishing what your why is for moving forward, you need to establish a clear identity for yourself.

Another key takeaway from James Clear's book is the idea of "stacking habits." I truly love this idea and have implemented this into my daily routine. Simply put (because I want you to buy his book) is that you currently have habits that come automatic to you. You make coffee the same way every day. You brush your teeth the same way. When you take a shower, you always wash your right shoulder first. (Got ya thinking about what you wash first in the shower didn't I?) Well what if you added some action that you want to become a habit right before or right after the habit you currently do. (I teased this idea in the chapter just before this one.) What if your intention is to add more movement into your day? Okay, easy. Make the coffee and while the coffee is brewing perform 20 push-ups. Do this same action day after day and a habit is formed.

2. Create a Positive Partnership with Food

Take a breath before eating anything and pause. What I am about to eat will stay inside of me for a long time. This food will either enhance or harm my wellbeing. If harm of any sort is on the menu, is it worth it? Think about food as a relationship, being mindful of the role that food has in the job of nourishing your body and mind. Think about where this food comes from. If it comes from a package or a box and has ingredients you don't recognize, then most likely your body won't recognize them either. If the food is of animal origin, what did that food have to go through to get to your plate? Try to steer in the direction of foods that are closest to the source of where they came from.

Ask yourself this question—What can I eat that has the best chance of enhancing my health? We make food choices all day long. So, take time to look at your options and make the best choice possible. Even fast-food restaurants now offer meatless burgers. Are they healthy? Probably too many additives and oil, but are they a better choice compared to their meat brother. At least for the environment and for the animal it is. Compare and then decide. Yes. Eat the meatless burger.

Have you heard of cognitive dissonance? Simply put, psychology.org refers to cognitive dissonance as "a situation involving conflicting attitudes, beliefs, or behaviors." For example, when people smoke (behavior) and they know that smoking causes cancer (cognition), they are in a state of cognitive dissonance. Knowing the benefits of eating whole food, plant-based foods, and then choosing to eat chicken fried steak and French fries is also an example of cognitive dissonance. We put good behavior on the back burner because we want instant gratification now not thinking of the consequences. Checking in with your food partnership before you take a bite will connect you with the big picture and hopefully trigger a behavioral change shift.

3. The Nutritional Gate Keeper

If you buy the food for you and your family, you are the nutritional gatekeeper. The nutritional gate keeper chooses what food makes it into the kitchen and ultimately what is consumed. This might be the biggest most important job you hold. Take your mind shift to the store with you. Think about it this way—the choices you make about what foods to feed you and your family will either promote or destroy health. It is that simple. If you have children, involve them in the shopping and preparing of the food. They are much more likely to buy in if they feel as if they have contributed to the effort.

Super family friendly meals include:

a. Burritos with veggies, brown rice, and beans.
b. Tacos with all the fixings where everyone can make their own.
c. Pizza with whole wheat pizza crust, tomato sauce, and veggies
d. Veggie soup and fresh, whole grain bread
e. Huge colorful salads with home-made salad dressing
f. Tofu scramble
g. Lasagna
h. Breakfast for dinner—groats or oatmeal with berries, almond butter, flax seed, nuts, shredded coconut
i. Nori rolls filled with rice and veggies (a great recipe is in the book by Ann Esselstyn, The Prevent and Reverse Heart Disease Cookbook).

j. Stuffed potatoes with nutritional yeast, veggies (can be found in the same cookbook above)

It doesn't matter if you have a family or are single—planning ahead is key to the grocery store trip.

Here is your action item list before going to the grocery store:

a. Create a simple meal plan for the week. Batch cook so that each meal carries over into 2-3 meals. Left overs are your best friend.

b. Use the Meal Planning Work Sheet below.

	Breakfast	Mid-Morning Snack	Lunch	Mid-Day Snack	Dinner
Monday					
Tuesday					
Wednesday					
Thursday					
Friday					
Saturday					
Sunday					

c. Take inventory of what you have and what you need and make a shopping list. This seems like a no-brainer, but how many times have you found yourself at the store not remembering what you already have and getting home and forgetting what you went to the store for in the first place?

d. You have heard this before, but do not go shopping hungry. Bad choices are made on an empty stomach. Eat something filling and healthy before venturing out to forage.

e. Take a reusable bag with you. You will save a tree, save money if you live in a state that charges for bags, but more importantly, there is nothing as sexy as a person carrying a reusable bag. Take my word for it. Gals and guys dig a reusable bag user. Using a reusable bag shows that you are conscientious, concerned about the environment (very hot), and that you think ahead. Our reusable bags of choice are the chicobag totes— Chicobags.com (https://chicobag.com/).

f. Choose wisely. What goes into your cart ends up eaten by someone you love. Everyone in the grocery store is checking out what everyone else is putting into their cart. Trust me, it's a thing. You are judged by the contents of your cart. If you have junk in your cart, it might be a signal to others that there is junk in your trunk, in your car, in your brain, and for sure in your body. Healthy foods in your cart are a clear signal to others that you are someone they want to hang out with.

g. Be a diligent food label sleuth. If you happen to pick up a package that has a food label, put it back. No, just kidding. While most items in your cart should be label free—whole-plant foods with minimal processing—there are certain items you do need that have a label. Always read the label first before committing it to your cart. Here are the basic guidelines to follow:

4. How to Read a Food Label Guidelines

First off—never believe the claims on the front of the box. They don't mean anything in the world of food labeling. Food manufacturers use suggestive wording to entice us to think that a packaged food is healthier than it is.

What does this mean?

a. Low Fat. This means that there is probably fat added to the food but also added sugar to replace additional fat that wasn't added on top of the fat that was already added.

b. Low Sugar or No Added Sugar. This may mean that sugar was added to the food or sugar substitutes were added to the food. This does not mean that the food is healthy.

c. Low Carb. What is a carb? Vegetables are carbs and so are potato chips. Just listing something as low carb means nothing and causes more harm than good. Classifying carbs as "bad" is ridiculous and uneducated. Simple carbohydrates void of nutrients are what we want to steer clear of, but not energy enhancing complex carbohydrates that fuel our bodies. When something states that it is "low carb," what is it high in? Probably added fat.

d. Multigrain / Made with Whole Grain. There is nothing here that says "100% whole grain." Multigrain just means that many grains (processed) are used and the term "made with whole grain" doesn't determine how much. Stating that the product has that ingredient in it without listing how much is saying nothing at all. Look for "100% whole grain," or put it back on the shelf.

e. Natural / Light. These terms sound all too good for us, but there are no requirements for the word natural or light to be on a label except for the fact that at some point there was something natural involved somewhere, or that there is a heavier version of the food-like product out there on some grocery store shelf. That there is an allowable amount of puss-in-milk is natural and acceptable. And cookies, cakes, and ice cream can be labeled "light." Don't buy into this marketing garbage.

f. Fortified / Enriched. Don't believe that just because a product is fortified or enriched that makes it healthy. Adding vitamins to junk still makes it junk—it just makes it enriched fortified junk.

g. Gluten Free. Because of food packaging and great marketing overnight, we all deemed gluten as the enemy, and we all had to run out and purchase only gluten-free items. What is gluten anyway? Gluten is a protein found in certain grains, and for most people, gluten is a very healthy addition to the diet. There are people who are sensitive to gluten and who choose alternative grains (grains with gluten include wheat, rye, spelt, and barley). Gluten-free does not mean healthy. It just means that gluten was removed, but what else was added?

h.   Fruit Flavored. Fruit flavored does not mean that there is any fruit in the product at all. It just means that a chemically engineered fruit flavoring of some sort has been added, and there is nothing healthy about that.

When you turn the box around to the nutritional fact label, look for a few bits of information:

a.   Serving size—compared to calorie count, this should be a lot.

b.   Calorie count—compared to serving size, this should a little.

c.   Ingredients you don't recognize—there shouldn't be any.

d.   Added fat—there shouldn't be any.

e.   Added salt—there shouldn't be any, and if there is, it should be low on the list. Less than a 1-1 ratio of calories to sodium.

f.   Added sugar—there shouldn't be any, and if there is, it should be low on the list. Watch out because food manufacturers can label sugar in many different ways. Look at all the various names for sugar including dextrose, fructose, galactose, glucose, lactose, maltose, sucrose, corn syrup, maltodextrin, and on and on and on.

5. Change Up the Landscape of Your Kitchen

Now that you are only bringing health-promoting food into your kitchen, let's take a quick snap shot of your kitchen. What lives on the counter? Whole food or packaged food? The counter is where the eye goes first, so the counter should display fruits and veggies of every type. Any processed packaged food should either be thrown away or stored away from view. This holds true also in the fridge. When you open your fridge, health should jump out at you. Your fridge should display a garden and not a morgue. Always have easy-to-grab healthy options for grab-and-goers. And don't hide these in the dark veggie drawer where no one ventures to go. These health-promoting foods should be front and center and easy to reach for.

In the "Staples and Shortcuts" chapter, you will get a tour of my kitchen and I will showcase all the must haves from brands to buy to appliances to own.

Do you own any cook books? Here are some great ones to consider. I have also included great reads that aren't necessarily cookbooks per se, but they include recipes in them.

a. *The How Not to Die Cookbook* by Michael Greger MD

b. *The Secrets to Ultimate Weight Loss: A revolutionary approach to conquer cravings, overcome food addiction, and lose weight without going hungry* by Chef AJ and Glen Merzer
c. *The Prevent and Reverse Heart Disease Cookbook: Over 125 Delicious, Life-Changing, Plant-Based Recipes* by Ann Crile Esselstyn and Jane Esselstyn
d. *Forks Over Knives—The Cookbook: Over 300 Recipes for Plant-Based Eating All Through the Year* by Del Sroufe
e. *Straight Up Food: Delicious and Easy Plant-based Cooking without Salt, Oil or Sugar* by Cathy Fisher
f. *Proteinaholic: How Our Obsession with Meat Is Killing Us and What We Can Do About It* by Garth Davis MD
g. *The Starch Solution* by John McDougall MD
h. *Power Foods for the Brain: An Effective 3-Step Plan to Protect Your Mind and Strengthen Your Memory* by Neal D. Barnard MD FACC

6. Cook and Eat at Home

There is nothing sexier than a man cooking in the kitchen—chopping fresh fruit for my hot oat groats for breakfast. Stir frying organic tofu and bok choy to go over the fresh homemade whole wheat toast I just pulled out of the oven for lunch. Stirring the hot pot full of simmering lentil stew for dinner. All the while, we are hanging out in the kitchen together. This is whole food, plant-based foreplay my friend. The way to the heart is to create beautiful culinary dishes together.

I am not talking about the BBQ. The act of barbequing actually, for me, is the least sexy thing a man can do. Think about it. First off you leave the kitchen where everyone is conjugating. Unless you have a very expensive appliance and ceiling hood to capture all that flying grease and animal goo, you are heading outside. Throwing dead animal flesh on a fire to watch fat drip all over the coals and then see those grill marks form is not sexy or manly in the least. And don't wear those grill marks as a badge of honor as those grill marks are actually heterocyclic amines—HCAs, which are known carcinogens that can contribute in the development of certain types of cancer. The National Institutes of Health (NIH) outlines HCAs and the cancer relationship as:

> HCAs form when amino acids (the building blocks of proteins and creatine, chemicals found in muscles) react at high cooking temperatures. Researchers have identified 17 different HCAs resulting from the cooking of muscle meats that may pose a human cancer risk.

Research conducted by the National Cancer Institute (NCI) as well as by Japanese and European scientists indicates that heterocyclic amines are created within muscle meats during most types of high-temperature cooking.

So, with barbequing off the menu, let's look at easy entry points for cooking at home.

Start with one meal per week and build up. Make a big pot of soup that cooks in less than an hour, and then you have left overs for days. Check out my favorite no-oil, no-animal-product, legume soup recipes in the recipe section. Depending on the soup, I use split peas, black beans for chili, and lentils. The great news is that if you are in a hurry, lentils are your go-to as they don't need any pre-soak time and they cook in one-third to one-half the time as beans. Bruce also has a great video on our website, onedaytowellness.org on how to prepare and cook beans called Bean Basics.

The key is to BATCH COOK. Time is always an issue and preparing food takes a back seat when other options are available. With Uber Eats now delivering disease-promoting McDonald's right to your front door, why would anyone spend their valuable time preparing food? I will tell you why. Because the trajectory of your entire life relies on you making health choices based on smarts and not on saving time, and saving a little time eating the standard American diet (SAD) food only slows you down in the long run. Believe me when I say that there is any place I would rather be than in a doctor's office. Shortcutting now on your health is actually a time suck and not a time saver in the productivity department. If time is an issue for you, batch cook. So simple.

As I showed you in the chapter before this one, "Taking Matters Literally into Your Own Hands," prep time is so minimal and will save you time and money. On Sunday morning soak a whole lotta beans and a whole lotta grains (check out my suggested bean and grain list in the recipes section). On Sunday night cook up both grains and beans. That night for dinner, you have all the fixings for a taco bar. Add fresh salsa, avocado, organic stone ground tortillas (that you toast up in your toaster), and you have created a Mexican restaurant right at home.

One last item about cooking and eating at home. Most restaurants are not in the business of providing health-promoting food. Restaurants want you to come back again and again. They cook with salt, sugar, and oil to optimize the taste of the food and just assume that the more salt, sugar, and oil the better. As you start eating whole food, plant-based without added SOS (salt, oil, sugar) you won't miss it, and actually, you will find that when you do go to a restaurant, the food will taste way too salty, sugary, and/or oily. You have control of your food when you cook at home. Cooking at home instead of eating out saves money and can save your life.

7. When Eating Out—Eat in First

Life happens, and we all have to eat out from time to time. Before you venture out to that restaurant or gathering where food is served, eat some wonderful soup, salad, veggies and hummus, or fruit. Drink a glass or two of water. This way you will be eating your greens and grains at home so that when you get to the restaurant, your stomach is already full of the good stuff so your decision making won't be clouded by your hunger. Hunger usually supersedes rational thought, and it gets even worse when there are tasty treats at every turn.

8. Change Your Idea of the "Snack"

The snack can make or break an otherwise health-promoting diet. When we are hungry, our willpower is little to none, and we are looking for whatever we can get our hands on quickly. We are not in the mood to prepare anything. This is where the food industry comes to the rescue. Food chemists know what we are craving. With the introduction of fast food and processed food, we have been programmed to reach for sugary, salty, and fatty foods that will immediately send dopamine to the pleasure center of our brain telling us to eat more and crave even more. Stopping this cycle is hard, but crucial in order to have our taste buds revert back to craving foods in their natural form. Chemists create food that highjacks our taste buds and that are void of nutrition, but foods that nature creates provides us with nutrition, energy, and life.

Here are my favorite, easy-to-prepare, delicious, nutritious, and energy-packed snacks. Have these pre-prepared and ready to grab and go. Keep them in your house, in your car, at the office, and in your pocket.

a. Dates and walnuts
b. Bananas with almond butter
c. Hummus (without oil) and whole grain toast
d. A bowl of berries or any fruit
e. Toaster toasted organic stone-ground corn tortillas
f. Seeds and dried fruits
g. Oatmeal with goji berries and flax seed

h. Carrots, celery, and salsa or hummus for dipping
i. Collard wrap with Mindy's Pesto
j. An entire cooked sweet potato
k. My black bean brownies
l. My chickpea cookies
m. My energy balls

9. Log Your Food with the Daily Dozen APP

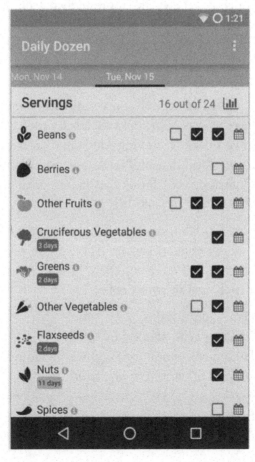

Download the APP "Dr. Greger's Daily Dozen." This is a free APP that lists the food you should be including in your diet every day for optimal health. It provides a description for each food, how many servings should be eaten, and a check off progress bar to encourage you to get your "Daily Dozen" in https://itunes.apple.com/us/app/dr.-gregers-daily-dozen/id1060700802?mt=8.

10. Download the 21-Day Vegan Kickstart APP at 21DayKickstart.org

This APP has everything you need from recipes to information about healthy eating. This free app is brought to you by The Physicians Committee for Responsible Medicine.

11. If you are a Dipper—Take Baby Steps.

In order to move in the right direction without fear of failure, some of us need to take baby steps. As mentioned earlier, one step that shows success will then lead to taking another step, and sooner than we know it, we have made our way up the staircase.

Here are a few examples of taking baby steps or dipping.

   a. Instead of half-and half in your coffee in the morning, try almond or soy or hemp or oat or cashew milk.
   b. Instead of a meat sandwich at lunch, try a veggie sandwich.
   c. Instead of an animal burger, try a veggie burger.

d.   Instead of a soda, try sparkling water with a small amount of fruit juice.

e.   Instead of a second cup of coffee, replace it with green tea.

f.   Instead of salted nuts, mix half salted with unsalted.

g.   Instead of an oil-based salad dressing, try balsamic vinegar with apple cider vinegar and Braggs Liquid Aminos.

h.   Instead of cheese, try nutritional yeast.

i.   Instead of meat, try mushrooms.

j.   Instead of ice cream, try frozen bananas.

k.   Instead of snacking on chips and crackers, try baby carrots, celery, and bell peppers.

11. Continue to Fill Your WHY Cup

Surround yourself with anything that will support your education and knowledge base. We have books on plant-based eating strategically placed all around our house, so when our guests happen to sit for some reason—the bathroom—there just happens to be fine reading material available. Subscribe to https://nutritionfacts.org/ where every day you receive information and research on plant-based choices so every day you are nudged in the right direction. Seek out others who are also on your same path to reinforce and assist you. In the Resources section, you will find additional material as this book is only scratching the surface on the science about the relationship between food and health.

The great news is—your taste buds heal. If you have been eating the standard American diet full of junk food and animal products, your taste buds have adjusted to craving these foods. These foods for the most part are loaded with added salt, sugar, and fat—way more than what is found in foods that nature has created. As you transition to healthier eating, your tastes will too. Yes, at first you will crave the foods you have been used to eating, but little by little you will shift to wanting more of the healthier options. Follow our 3G eating advice, and you will not feel deprived. Remember, with 3G you are always able to eat the foods you love. You are just eating the most health-promoting foods first. As you travel along this path, you will start to prefer the healthier alternatives because your taste buds heal.

TAKEAWAY TIPS

Transitioning from eating food that harms to one that heals takes a mind shift. Knowing the why and then implementing the how is difficult but doable. Identifying if you are a dipper or diver will help set the road map of how to process and then proceed.

1. Implement the 3G eating strategy to feel satiated and not deprived as you transition.

2. Plan ahead. Prepare ahead—from meal planning to shopping to storage.
3. Arm yourself with all the information you can knowing that the more you stick to the plan the easier it will become. Taste buds do heal and food that nature provides tastes amazing if we give our taste buds time to recalibrate.

PENIS TIP –
HOW'S IT HANGIN'?

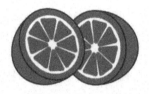

I am not insinuating in any way that I was promiscuous growing up in the 70s. Let's just say that I was totally monogamous quite a few times. That being said, I saw quite a few variations of penises and the way of the hang. Some totally normal and some downright scary. Thank goodness my current monogamy of close to 40 years has stuck, and the hang is just fine. I will leave it at that.

In the article "Top 10 things you didn't know about your penis," written by Tim Newman, Feb. 8, 2018 for *Medical News Today,* one of the interesting facts that was highlighted was the degree in which the penis "hung" erect. This varies from penis to penis. And there is no wrong or right way to hang.

The flaccid penis can fall varying degrees to the right or the left. There is no right or wrong way to fall. And an erect penis can point in a multitude of directions as well.

This article even included a comparison chart if you would like to measure your erect penis to see where you fall or point—literally.

Zero degrees represents when the penis points straight up toward your nose and 90 degrees points straight out at your partner. Isn't this amazing, interesting information? Of the men measured here are the stats. How do you measure up?

4.9% of men pointed between 0-30 degrees
29.6% of men pointed between 30-60 degrees
30.9% of men pointed between 60-85 degrees
9.9% of men pointed between 85-95 degrees
19.8% of men pointed between 95-120 degrees
4.9% of men pointed between 120-180 degrees

PENIS PALS AND PARTNER POINTERS

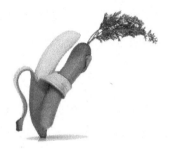

Be the change you wish to see in the world.

Ghandi

Love doesn't make the world go around. Love is what makes the ride worthwhile.

— Franklin P. Jones

Penis Pals

I t is not only how you hang, but who you hang out with that says a whole lot about your health. Surrounding yourself with like-minded health conscious pals does wonders for all aspects of your life. As Dan Buettner, author of *The Blue Zones* states, "Select your friendships carefully. Gather people around you who will reinforce your lifestyle. The people you surround yourself with influence your behaviors, so choose friends who have healthy habits." And then be an outstanding role model for others.

Bruce and I live by Gandhi's words, "Be the change you wish to see in the world." If you don't, then who will? Don't wait for someone else to change their behavior before you change yours. Be the leader for positive change.

What if one partner is on board but the other is not? This is hard, and it doesn't make staying on course easy in any way. Although we can't change anyone else's behavior, we can nudge. Not by pushing, shaming, or blaming, but by lovingly steering the conversation. Here are a few ideas to try:

1. Offer to cook a new recipe for your partner. What does he/she love to eat? It is easy to search for a plant based, no-oil option. Find a recipe your partner will love, and try plant-based substitutes for their animal counter parts.
2. How about:
   a. Jackfruit to replace pork in BBQ pulled pork burgers.

b. Soy Curls to replace chicken in chicken stir fry.

c. Nutritional Yeast instead of cheese on top of salads or on popcorn.

d. Plant milk to replace cow milk for coffee, cereal, baked goods.

e. Beans, lentils, and peas to replace meat in soups, stews, or taco bars.

f. Tofu or flax eggs (see my recipe in recipe section) instead of eggs for baking or French toast.

g. Frozen bananas instead of ice cream to dip into dark chocolate pudding or to make soft serve.

h. Date sugar to replace cane sugar for anytime you need a sweetener.

i. Cacao instead of cocoa for anytime that needs a chocolatey taste.

j. Dark chocolate instead of milk chocolate because dark chocolate is delicious and loaded with antioxidants without the animal milk or butter fat.

3. Share a documentary together based on plant-based nutrition. Try *Forks Over Knives, Cowspiracy, Game Changers, The Truth About Your Food with FOOD, INC., What the Health, Super Size Me.*

4. Shop together in the grocery store or better yet at the Farmers Market so you can shake the hand of the person who grew that food. By choosing living, colorful, nutritious food that wasn't stressed or harmed, you are opening the door to compassion, empathy, and thoughtfulness.

The best you can do is to lead by example. Once you KNOW you can't UNKNOW. It is easier to make the plant-based food and stick to your guns when you are aware of the detriments of making ill-informed or uneducated decisions. Knowing that animal products can clog the arteries that then can lead to ED and possibly death might make one pause and choose something less disease promoting and more health promoting. Your partner might not be there yet, but if you lead by example with small loving nudges, he/she may follow. The key is to pull your partner in and not push him/her away. Leading by example is looking at the end game. If the end game is a great robust sex life, then choosing plant-based looks pretty good.

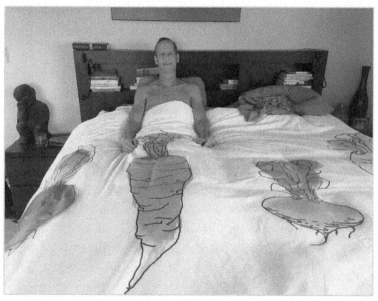

Our lead-by example bedspread

Partner Pointers for a Healthy Libido

Thich Nhat Hanh outlines in his book, *How to Love,* that there are four elements of true love. They are loving kindness, compassion, joy, and equanimity.

Being happily married for almost 40 years, business partners for 20, parents to three boys, and living in the size of a tin can together for three years, I am often asked the question, "What's your secret?" We don't have just one secret. We love kindly. We are compassionate to each other. We show our joy in all the little things. And we practice equanimity meaning an inclusive shared life. There are many linked actions we perform that create calm, peace, and balance. A beautiful, playful dance from honest meaningful interaction and connection leads to deep intimacy and passion that follows.

Here are my top "12 Partner Pointers" for you to ponder. Many of these pointers validate what you already do or know you should do, but for whatever reason, they aren't part of your current repertoire. Try one or two or all 12 and see if these lead to a libido boost for both of you. This list has worked for us.

1. Face your partner when you talk to him or her with nothing in between you. This means turning your entire body flush with theirs. Body language is as/or more important than what you are actually saying. Show your partner you care with your actions first and lean in.

2. In a conversation, cut out distractions. Close your computer and turn off the phone and TV. Let

your partner know that he/she is the most important person in your life and nothing is more precious than your time together.

3. Listen more than talk. Ask questions that are relevant, nonjudgmental, and continue the flow of the conversation with honest input. Praise your partner's accomplishments and laugh at his/her jokes, but also offer constructive feedback if it is warranted. Be there for it all, not just when it is easy.

4. Be unexpected. Do a chore that normally your partner does. Bring home a gift or small token of appreciation. Write your partner a love note. Hand your partner a towel as he/she comes out of the shower. Get up earlier than your partner and have coffee ready. Better yet, bring him/her coffee in bed. These small gestures are what your partner will remember all day long.

5. Cook and eat together at home. There is something very special and sexual about cooking together. Shift the mind set from, "It takes too much time, and it would be much easier to go out to eat" to "Together we will plan, then prepare, this glorious delicious food and sit down and eat what we made. We will share our culinary creation, discussing the aroma, texture, taste, and presentation." Even if you don't like to cook, find one dish that you would be willing to make. Julia Child tells us, *"I think careful cooking is love,*

don't you? The loveliest thing you can cook for someone who's close to you is about as nice a valentine as you can give."

6. After dinner, take a walk together. Research shows that moving after a meal helps with the digestive process. The evening walk together is actually Bruce's and my favorite time together. We hold hands, discuss everything or nothing. It doesn't really matter. It is this time of day where the day has settled down, and calm has set in. This time of the day is exhale time for us and in the exhale, one finds calm and connection.

7. Be honest (when I read this section to Bruce his input was, "add NO CHEATING ON YOUR SPOUSE"). I will keep it at "Be honest." This is THE best gift you can give your loved one. I know that Bruce would never be dishonest or keep anything from me. This truth sets both of us free. There is no wondering "what if" or wasted energy spent on being jealous. Early on in our marriage, it was actually a running joke that Bruce could never have an affair because I used up all his energy already, and it would be too much trouble to handle another relationship.

8. Only purchase what you can pay off at the end of the month. Financial stress can squelch any romantic moment. If you are worried about how to pay your bills, that is all that is on your mind and everything else takes a back seat. Don't let

these financial hardships be self-inflicted. Bruce and I, early on in our relationship, went without on many occasions just because we didn't want to be in debt. My engagement ring cost $200.00. That was what we could afford without financing. We always bought used cars, and today we only own one car. But we do own two bicycles. We go to bed at night free from debt and free from having the worry of how are we going to pay for the "stuff." Stuff doesn't add anything to a relationship. Being debt-free is the best investment you can make in a relationship.

I actually wrote about stuff in one of my past blogs:

The Powers and Perils of STUFF

The beauty of living in an RV is that the stuff you carry has to be limited. Our RV is a V8. This means that everything we lug around in the RV adds to the load that we lug. At six-to-eight miles a gallon, every pound adds up to the overall cost of fueling our nonprofit mission. This blog is to discuss our stuff and how less stuff allows us to live free.

There are three types of stuff:
1. Utility Stuff
2. Recall Stuff
And
3. Status Stuff

Utility stuff is stuff we need to do the stuff we love to do. Bruce is an avid surfer, and he needs LOTS of surf boards for the variety of size and strength of the wave he is facing. He relies on his quiver to allow him to surf whatever wave presents itself on a given day.

Recall Stuff is to savor the memories of time. Don't judge me, but my mom had, for as long as I can remember, a dental bridge she wore that contained five false teeth. My mom died almost 20 years ago, but I still have her bridge. It is tucked up in a cabinet in my house in a box labeled "mom" and, among many other memories of my mom, those teeth are there to stay. For no reason and for every reason, I cannot part with my mom's teeth.

Status Stuff is what many of us accumulate for no reason other than to satisfy our desire to be IN. What others think of us plays a huge role in the stuff that surrounds us. We "dress to impress." We drive the cool car to "be seen." Our choices are based on what is deemed "correct" and "in keeping" and "status quo." It is easier to move in the direction of the tide than fight against it.

Utility Stuff check. When we moved into the RV, I stocked our cabinets with stuff that was 100 percent essential, and included only the essentials in clothing, and, yes, surf boards and wet suits just in case there is an ocean on either coast that shows a wave or two. I stocked work items, and all that we need to eat and thrive nutritionally.

Recall Stuff check. What recall stuff did make it into the RV? No, my mom's teeth did not make the cut. A sweet pillow with the picture of our three boys did, however, and I look at it every day reminding me of how amazingly lucky I am to have three wonderful sons.

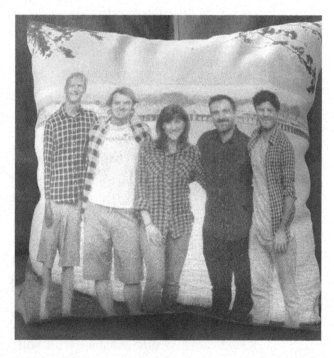

Other than that, all memories of the past are tucked away at our house in California as Bruce and I create new memories on the road. And these memories are not captured by acquiring more stuff. They are memories that we tuck in our hearts.

9. Prioritize your time. We are all so busy. No matter if we are single, coupled, or have a family, a common theme is that there is always something needed to be done. Our days are full of "must do's." These "must do's" warrant our time and have to get done. Then there are "want to do's." These are the things that we GET to do. These are the nuggets of time that bring us pleasure and joy. Get the "must do's" done but then decide what is truly worthy to make it on to your "Get to do" list. Is watching TV, playing a video game, or perusing social media after dinner worthy or is going for a walk with your partner or family more worthy and worthwhile? Ask yourself this question, "Is what I am about to spend my time on have the potential of creating a lifelong lasting memory?" If the answer is no, then perhaps search out something that will. Life is only a bunch of moments linked together, creating memories for us to paint our landscape. I don't want to let moments pass by unnoticed or unused. I want a life tapestry full of all the colors of the rainbow.

10. Keep your expectations in check. Christmas was a big deal in my house as I was growing up. Lots of extended family. Lots of food, and most of all, lots of presents. Lots and Lots of presents. My

first Christmas with Bruce was no different. I bought him—I think looking back now—around ten presents and had an overstuffed stocking waiting for him Christmas morning. I was so excited for the gift exchange to begin. Here it comes, my first gift. A beautiful watch. I love it. Okay, ready for my next gift. I sat there stunned. There was only one gift, and no overstuffed stocking. This was not my expectation of Christmas. I tried to put on a "I am not disappointed because all I got was one gift when you still have nine to open and an overstuffed stocking" face, but I didn't do a very good job of it. I loved my watch; don't get me wrong—but I had lived 21 years prior with lots and lots of gifts to open and this Christmas was shattering because all my expectations were not being met.

It took me putting on my big-girl pants and spending a lot of time within my own head to determine why I had these expectations, and if there was going to be a relationship with this man, should I be the one to change my expectations or should he? It was going to be me. That Christmas I learned that holding expectations of what you want the outcome to be is setting you up for the worst outcome. Having realistic expectations eliminates disappointment.

There are major expectations I have for Bruce. He must be forever faithful, dependable, and honest. If these expectations are met, then I am good with one gift and to hell with a stocking at Christmas.

11. Play and have fun. Just yesterday Bruce and I were having lunch at our favorite local Santa Cruz salad bar and this woman came up to us and asked, "Excuse me, but are you dating?" I said, "Only for the past 40 years." She laughed and then got serious, "Are you saying you have been married for that long? I thought you were dating because you are having such fun with each other and you are so cute together." She congratulated us and on she went. This is not the first time this has happened to us. We really enjoy each other's company, and I guess this shows. We joke and laugh out loud in public. We touch each other in nuanced ways. We treat each other as pal and partner. We have not lost our sense of courtship playfulness. And why would we? And why should you?

12. What drives YOU? I saved this one for last, as this one is where many couples get into trouble. When one partner finds his/her passion or has an interest that is all consuming, the other partner may feel pushed aside, feel less important, feel overshadowed, even resentful, and may be jealous of this activity and how much time it is taking away from the relationship. Resentment builds, and the relationship suffers.

What if the opposite were to be the case?

What if the activity energizes and sparks passion into the relationship? Stay with me and I will try to explain. When I was competing for the National Aerobic Championship Title, I was all consumed. My time was either spent physically preparing my body or mentally training my mindset. Bruce had no idea what I was doing and had absolutely no interest. He did, however, see how driven I was and how focused I was and would repeatedly tell me how proud he was of me for my motivation and drive. The focus and commitment I had was contagious. I felt so good about my progression and my sense of accomplishment that I was excited about everything else in my life. My passion fueled me, and that in turn fueled our relationship. I made it my mission to include my family in the process and not exclude them. (It would have been easier to do the latter.) I made it a priority to carve out quality time for each of them—at that time Bruce and I had our relationship to care for and two small boys to nurture as well.

To accomplish this monumental feat, I took a page out of a man's playbook and compartmentalized. Women (I am not including all women, just me and all women I know) have a very difficult time doing this as we are multi taskers. We try to do everything at once. We are quite good at performing many tasks at the same time, but trying to master all, we fall short at doing them all well. We get them done, but at the expense of our sanity. This is totally not our fault. We are, as a sex, expected to do it all so we hunker down and do our best.

My observation has been that men have the amazing talent of working on one task at a time and not letting other tasks interfere with the task at hand. Take—the orgasm. I think this is why men have no trouble having an orgasm quickly. They are focused on only one thing. Men—I will let you in on a secret. Women—try as we may not to do so—we multitask during sex. We try so hard to think of only what is happening at the moment, but our minds don't work the same way yours does. We are in the moment, but then we are thinking about work. Nope, we are back in the moment. Oh, there we go again—now we are thinking about the laundry that is in the washer needing to go into the dryer. Okay, we are back. Oh, shit—there we go again. When is my dentist appointment next week? And back and forth until finally we squeak out an orgasm. This isn't our fault either. It is how we are wired. Now, this isn't all women, but if you are a woman reading this, I bet ten bucks you can relate on some level.

Bruce actually has an alternative view on the orgasm event. He thinks it has to do with how beautifully nature has designed us. Nature wants men to orgasm quickly so that our species perpetuates. A women's ability to have an

123

orgasm or not is irrelevant to the grand plan. All that matters is that the sperm and egg hook up. The rest is inconsequential.

Anyway, back to the "What drives You" thought—I digress. Having your own thing that drives you and that in turn drives the relationship is key to "keeping it all together." By compartmentalizing, I was able to "shelf" the all-consuming aspect of my activity and only bring to the partnership table the energy that the passion pushed. No resentment from Bruce, just a whole lotta "Wow, whatever she is doing over in that other world, keep doing it because it sure does bring light over here." Our "own thing" drives us, differentiates us, identifies us, energizes us. This should also fuel and connect all other aspects of our lives and not separate us from them.

TAKEAWAY TIPS

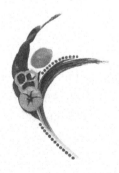

The relationship you nurture with your partner has to be on the top of your priority list. A healthy sex life is a by-product of a healthy relationship and not the other way around. Put the work in and you will be rewarded in every way. The tips from this chapter are all takeaways and are consequential, so do keep them in mind.

1. Be present and available.
2. Be honest and open.
3. Have fun.

PENIS TIP – MASTURBATION LEADS TO....

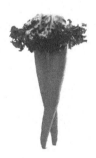

My father provided words of great wisdom as I was growing up. He would quote my grandmother who always told him that if he played with himself, he would walk backwards. This was a joke that I had to endure over and over as more times than not my dad would walk around the house backwards. "Ha, I get it, Dad. Now stop already."

You may have heard that masturbation can cause blindness, hairy palms, impotence, cancer, acne, and a myriad of other diseases/disorders. Even Dr. Kellogg created a cereal he thought would curb the behavior. Yes, the Kellogg's corn flake was thought to possess anti-masturbation properties (I can't make this stuff up) because of its bland flavor. John Harvey Kellogg was born in 1852. He invented Corn Flakes in 1878 in the hope that plain food would stop people from masturbating. Mr. Kellogg, the man who created Corn Flakes, produced the cereal in the late 19th century and marketed it as a "healthy, ready-to-eat anti-masturbatory morning meal."

Nothing could be further from the truth.

> Masturbation once thought evil and the cause of many diseases has been proven medically not to cause mental illness, physical weakness, or any type of disease or death; it is a normal aspect of human sexual development.

> — Domeena C. Renshaw on Eric.ed.gov

Actually, mutual masturbation can lead to an open, loving exchange and increase erectile function. Learning what turns on your partner can be a powerful aphrodisiac all by itself. A 2015 study on the Role of Masturbation in Marital and Sexual Satisfaction showed that the female "masturbators had significantly more orgasms, greater sexual desire, higher self-esteem, and greater marital and sexual satisfaction, and required less time to sexual arousal."

WORKING OUT AND WORKING IN

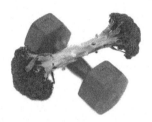

Now that you have all that energy—Move Man!!!

Do the best you can until you know better.
Then when you know better, do better.

— Maya Angelou

The WORK OUT

As discussed, erectile dysfunction can stem from many contributing factors—obesity, high cholesterol, diabetes, high blood pressure, even depressions and medication side effects. Even sitting on a bike seat for too long can cause the woodie to wilt. But as also discussed, when you treat the root cause, the symptoms get better or cease to exist.

One amazing side effect of better health is an explosion of energy. This may be that you have included exercise into your daily routine from the get go and you are seeing that you can do more than ever before or, now that you are feeling better, you want to add exercise into the mix. How you fuel yourself should always be on the top of your priority list, but exercise and moving more throughout the day is right up there.

For exercise tips you have come to the right chapter. Not only am I the proud mom and wife of great penises, but I am also the creator of both The Gliding Discs and Tabata Bootcamp. Heck, I was even the 1991 World Aerobic Champion. I have been lecturing on the fitness and wellness circuit for over 35 years, have over 500 fitness videos under my belt, and have seen every fitness trend come and go and come back again. I am about to get geeky here, but the more you know about what you are choosing to do, the more you will adhere.

Let's discuss first the exercise selection you should be including into your fitness training, and then I offer up a few personalized plans based on time and preference.

A well-rounded exercise routine should include steady-state training, interval training in the form of HIIT (High Intensity Interval Training), strength training, and some form of stretching. All these can easily be incorporated over a series of days. The body also needs time for recovery and repair. Recovery is as important as work, and this recovery component is many times overlooked when someone is just starting an exercise routine because they want to see results quickly. This can lead to overuse and injury, so how you schedule these trainings into your days is important to the overall sustainability of the routine.

Steady-State Training

Steady-state cardio may be defined as any form of aerobic training where your heart rate is elevated to anywhere between 135 to 150 beats per minute (this could be higher or lower depending on the individual) and held there for a period of 30 to 60 minutes. It is important to add some sort of steady-state training at least once to twice a week in order to maintain baseline aerobic steady-state fitness. This can be as easy as adding in a long walk, sustained low-intensity run, cardio-fitness class, or swim. Any activity that maintains the heart rate at 60-75% of VO2 max is appropriate.

Interval Training

Interval training can be described as discontinuous aerobic activity. Any activity that mixes lower and higher intensity intervals can be defined as interval training. Interval training can alternate between lower aerobic and higher aerobic activity (oxygen dependent) or between aerobic and anaerobic activity (oxygen independent).

High Intensity Interval Training (HIIT)

HIIT is an interval-based training protocol that has shown great success in the fitness gain and weight loss story. HIIT typically consists of 20 minutes or less of training time. HIIT training focuses on exercises that use major muscle groups (largest most blood flow demanding muscles—gluts, quads, hams), compound movement (multi-joint movement meaning hip, knee, and ankle) and high intensity training. HIIT training taps the energy sources inside the muscle.

The reason why HIIT works better for fat loss than steady state training is this: When you do a cardio session at the same pace for the entire workout duration, your body goes into what is called a steady state. This means that your body has adjusted itself to the intensity you are going and tries hard to conserve energy (calories).

With steady-state training, you are also not creating a "state of disruption" for the body, so recovery time for steady-state is relatively short. Conversely, with HIIT, the body works at its hardest, and it needs to use energy (calories) to repair itself post exercise. This is where the difference is evident with HIIT. In the post workout recovery, the body's metabolism remains elevated for hours, burning additional calories. This is called the afterburn or EPOC (Excess Post-exercise Oxygen Consumption). Research has shown that the most amount of post workout afterburn happens within the first 1-2 hours after the workout is completed but can continue at low levels up to 24 hours.

EPOC

Excess Post-exercise Oxygen Consumption (EPOC) is the amount of oxygen consumed by the body after exercise is completed. Research has shown this accelerates weight loss. EPOC consumes oxygen at an elevated rate, as well as expending energy at an elevated rate, by the following methods:

1. Replenishment for the immediate source of energy known as the phosphate system. The body is also restoring the muscle glycogen that has been consumed during exercise.
2. The body continues to expend energy post-exercise to re-oxygenate the blood. During post exercise, the body restores levels of circulatory hormones to normal.
3. During EPOC, the body expends energy to cool off after exercise.
4. Energy is consumed at an elevated rate to return the body to a normal breathing and heart rate.

Evidence suggests that high intensity interval RESISTANCE training has a more pronounced effect on EPOC levels than similar types of aerobic training. Additionally, current research indicates that as resistance intensity increases, the EPOC duration also increases. In a 2011 study, one six-minute workout bout produced five times the calorie burn after the workout was over. The calories burned during the six-minute workout were 50 calories and the metabolism remained elevated for 24 hours burning an additional 250 calories. This total of 300 calories is comparable to what people typically burn during 30 minutes of steady state exercise.

In summary, intermittent high-intensity resistance training appears to have the greatest effect on EPOC. Weight-loss benefits of EPOC for men and women participating in resistance exercise occur over a prolonged time period, since calories are expended at a low rate in post exercise. However, body fat loss is typically higher for HIIT resistance training programs as compared to steady-state only based programs.

All interval training has bouts of work and rest. The ratio of the work to rest provides either enough rest, just enough rest, or not enough rest to then go into the rest-work bout. Positive recovery interval training is when the work bout is greater or equal to the rest bout.

Examples of this Positive recovery timing are:
30 seconds work / 30 seconds rest
60 seconds work / 75 seconds rest
20 seconds work / 40 seconds rest

Negative Recovery interval training is when the work bout is greater than the rest bout. Examples of this timing are:

30 seconds work / 20 seconds rest
20 seconds work / 10 seconds rest
60 seconds work / 40 seconds rest

Here are some variations of HIIT that are tried, tested, and tough.

Fartlek Training

Fartlek training, created in Sweden in the 1940s incorporates usually, but not limited to, bouts of interval slower to faster running. Fartlek translated means "speed play." The timing with Fartlek training is not a set time but more irregular in its lengths and speeds compared with other forms of interval training. Here an example of Fartlek training. The suicide drill where you run as hard as you can to a short destination —approximately 10 seconds away—then walk back. Now run to a destination slightly further away—20 seconds and walk back. Repeat 6-10 times, increasing the distance each time.

Sprint Interval Training

Sprint training is similar to Fartlek but doesn't vary the distance. Sprint interval training is referred to as "Walk back sprinting" which is running for a short distance and then walking back to the starting point and then repeated at the same or a varied distance. This provides for just enough recovery to be able to repeat the interval.

Tabata Timing

Tabata timing was first researched in 1996 by Isumi Tabata in Japan. This is a HIIT that is only four minutes in duration. The timing is 20 seconds on and 10 seconds off— a true negative recovery. The 20 seconds are all out to failure and the 10 seconds are full recovery. This is repeated 8 times to equal 4 minutes.

30-20-10

I like to refer to this HIIT as hard, harder, hardest. For 30 seconds, work at a comfortable yet challenging pace.

For the next 20 seconds increase the intensity so that you are breathing hard but still doable. The last 10 seconds is an all-out effort to failure. Repeat this pattern 4-10 times.

Having these timing protocols in your exercise toolbox, you have unlimited workouts to choose from. Below are valuable considerations and a few work-out plans to choose from or to provide you with information to create your own. If you already have an exercise routine, see if you are incorporating a variety in the mix for maximum success. Also below are suggestions for how to make your workouts the best they can be. *Always check with your doctor before starting an exercise routine.*

When adding HIIT to your training routine here are some considerations:

1. HIIT should not be scheduled on consecutive days, as this type of training requires the highest intensity effort. Muscles need to replenish and rest. This workout protocol is best practiced 2-3 days per week.

2. Prepare for the intensity with a positive mental mindset. Research studies suggest that a person's mental mindset plays a key role in their outcome of their efforts. Commit to the work and the work will pay you back.

3. Always keep the body guessing—change up the routine often. Every workout will challenge and excite various muscle and movement patterns.

4. Include a warm up and cool down.

5. Vary the time of work-to-rest intervals. Choose from a multiple research proven timing and work to rest ratios 40/30/20, 30/20/10, 20/10 listed above.

Workout Plan #1

You have 30-60 minutes a day to exercise. Below is a sample week of workout suggestions along with two sample HIIT workouts for you to try. If you are new to all this, don't worry as I have loaded the backend support for this book for you. For exercise and more sample workout ideas go to onedaytowellness.org or just Google my name (Mindy Mylrea) and hundreds of my workouts will pop up.

Monday

30-60 minute HIIT workout incorporating both cardio and strength

Sample HIIT circuit line up using only body weight

30 minutes HIIT circuit—20/10 Timing and 30/20/10 Timing

Warmup	5 minutes total body movement including jogging, squatting, lunging, sitting and standing, twisting, bending		
Timing	**30 Sec**	**20 Sec**	**10 Sec**
Exercise	Lower Body Lunge back with right leg	Lower Body Lunge back with right leg and jump	Lower Body Lunge back with right leg and jump keeping right leg in air on lunge back like you are kicking open a door behind you.
	Lower Body Same with left leg	Lower Body Same with left leg	Lower Body Same with left leg
	Upper Body Push-up	Upper Body Tricep push-up	Upper Body Chest and Tricep push-up
	Upper Body Hold Hand Plank	Upper Body Move from hand plank to elbow plank and back again	Upper Body Repeat with push-up at hand plank
	Core Supine bridge to seated V sit	Core Supine bridge twist to seated V sit	Core V sit hold and torso twist
	Core Prone down dog to plank	Core Add one leg pull in to chest	Core Add twist to leg pull into chest
Timing	20-10 Timing Tabata Squat Jumps		
Repeat the same 30-20-10 timing exercises again			

Timing	30 Sec	20 Sec	10 Sec
Exercise	Lower Body Lunge back with left leg	Lower Body Lunge back with left leg and jump	Lower Body Lunge back with left leg and jump keeping left leg in air on lunge back like you are kicking open a door behind you.
	Lower Body Same with right leg	Lower Body Same with right leg	Lower Body Same with right leg
	Upper Body Push-up	Upper Body Tricep push-up	Upper Body Chest and Tricep push-up
	Upper Body Hold Hand Plank	Upper Body Move from hand plank to elbow plank and back again	Upper Body Repeat with push-up at hand plank
	Core Supine bridge to seated V sit	Core Supine bridge twist to seated V sit	Core V sit hold and torso twist
	Core Prone down dog to plank	Core Add one leg pull in to chest	Core Add twist to leg pull into chest
Timing	20-10 Timing Tabata Burpees and alternating jump lunges		
Cool down and stretch - 5 minutes			

Tuesday

60-90 minutes of steady state cardio.

Wednesday

30-60 minute HIIT workout incorporating both cardio and strength.

Thursday

60-90 minutes of steady state cardio.

Friday

30-60 minute HIIT workout incorporating both cardio and strength.

Sample HIIT circuit line up using only hand weights

30 minutes HIIT circuit—20/10 Timing and 30/20/10 Timing

For 60-minute circuit—repeat all

Warmup	5 minutes- total body movement including jogging, squatting, lunging, sitting and standing, twisting, bending		
Timing	**30 Sec**	**20 Sec**	**10 Sec**
Exercise	Lower Body Holding weights, step up onto bench with one leg	Lower Body Without weights, step up onto bench and jump	Lower Body Increase depth of landing and height of jump
	Lower Body Same with other leg	Lower Body Same with other leg	Lower Body Same with other leg
	Upper Body Laying on bench - Supine chest press with weights - full range of motion	Upper Body Supine chest press with weights - half range of motion	Upper Body Supine chest press with weights. Cross weights at full extension
	Upper Body Bent over Row - full range of motion	Upper Body Bent over Row - half range of motion	Upper Body Bent over Row - cross weights at full extension
	Core V sit with weights held at chest	Core V sit with weights twist torso	Core V sit hold with feet off floor
	Core Plank with hands on weights	Core Alternate lifting weight to side plank	Core Add twist under torso
Timing	20-10 Timing Tabata Alternate lunging to side holding hand weights		
Repeat the same 30-20-10 timing exercises again			

Timing	30 Sec	20 Sec	10 Sec
Exercise	Lower Body Holding weights step up onto bench with one leg	Lower Body Without weights step up onto bench and jump	Lower Body Increase depth of landing and height of jump
	Lower Body Same with other leg	Lower Body Same with other leg	Lower Body Same with other leg
	Upper Body Laying on bench - Supine chest press with weights - full range of motion	Upper Body Supine chest press with weights - half range of motion	Upper Body Supine chest press with weights Cross weights at full extension
	Upper Body Bent over Row - full range of motion	Upper Body Bent over Row - half range of motion	Upper Body Bent over Row - cross weights at full extension
	Core V sit with weights held at chest	Core V sit with weights twist torso	Core V sit hold with feet off floor
	Core Plank with hands on weights	Core Alternate lifting weight to side plank	Core Add twist under torso
Timing	20-10 Timing Tabata Twisted squat jumps and Star Jacks		
Cook down and stretch - 5 minutes			

Saturday

Long walk

Sunday

Yoga, stretch or some form of mind body movement

The WORK IN

Take a step back in history to pre computer, pre junk food, pre health club on every corner, and we will see very little obesity, much less chronic disease, and better health over all. Tell a pioneer from 200 years ago that in the 2020s we would be overfed and undernourished, and they would have thought you were crazy. Tell a parent in 1960 that if they were raising their family today, their child would be at risk for obesity, Type 2 diabetes, an early death, and not to mention erectile dysfunction. They would have not believed you.

Well here we are in the 2020s, and one thing is for sure. The rise of health clubs and fitness studios is not making a dent in the obesity epidemic. On the contrary, the health club market is growing at the same rate as the obesity crisis. We are actually moving less instead of more, and thinking that a one-hour trip to the gym will fix an otherwise sedentary day. Well unfortunately the opposite is true.

I have spent my entire adult career teaching fitness instructors and personal trainers how to teach fitness. I am proud of what I have contributed. But it has been only in the last ten years have I combined fitness with food. Food is the most important piece and moving throughout the day is next in line. The workout routine, as I have outlined above, is very important, but if you are not moving throughout the day, then you are missing the message. The people who live the longest and thrive move naturally all day long. They can easily sit and stand on and off the floor. They can twist, turn, and rotate without aches and pains. They incorporate what us fitness folk call functional movement—movement we use during everyday living. The fitness industry's message has resonated the same tenet for years—Spend one hour at the gym and all will be well. One hour of exercise 3-4 days a week will fix all life's idle tendencies. Not so according to numerous research studies.

In one 2012 analysis that looked at the results from 18 studies, it was found that those who sat for the longest periods of time were twice as likely to have diabetes or heart disease compared to those who sat less.

The analysis also showed that an exercise routine (the typical work OUT) doesn't counteract the damage incurred by prolonged daily sitting. All that time spent in the gym doesn't make up for the rest of the day if the rest of the day is spent sitting. The studies point to just moving, staying active as the critical component for becoming and staying functionally fit.

As reported by USA Today:

> The risk of heart failure was more than double for men who sat for at least five

hours a day outside of work and didn't exercise very much compared with men who were physically active and sat for less than two hours a day. The risk was lowest for men who exercised the most and sat for fewer than two hours a day.

Government statistics show almost half of the people report sitting more than six hours a day, and 65 percent say they spend more than two hours a day watching TV. "If you've been sitting for an hour, you've been sitting too long," says James Levine, co-director of Obesity Solutions at Mayo Clinic in Phoenix/Scottsdale, Arizona State University.

What is most alarming is that the studies also show that a regular fitness routine does NOT counteract the effects of prolonged sitting. This study that followed more than 82,000 men for 10 years found that these risk factors were present no matter how much they exercised. Hopefully you are reading this standing up!

Why is it that sitting is so detrimental to our health? A study from NASA explains that the body deteriorates at a faster pace in an anti-gravity environment. Sitting for an extended period of time replicates this environment. Poor sitting techniques can create ever more issues. Esther Gokhale, creator of the Gokhale Method and a posture expert, writes:

> In our stack sitting method (which is really healthy sitting, primal sitting, if you will),

you have your behind out behind, but not exaggeratedly. That's very important. Then your bones stack well and the muscles alongside your spine are able to relax... Now when you breathe, your whole spine lengthens and settles, lengthens and settles. There's this movement which stimulates circulation and allows natural healing to be going on as you sit.

If you sit poorly, whether relaxed and slumped or upright and tense, you've lost all of that. So do we want to blame [all the adverse health effects] on sitting, or do we want to blame it on the poor sitting form? That's my question.

My thought is that how we sit and how long we sit both are key to our longevity. My motto is, "Stand instead of sit, sway instead of stand, walk instead of sway, and run instead of walk." Bruce and I try to find every opportunity to move functionally. We have a very long staircase in our house that leads to the upper level where the living quarters and kitchen are. In our RV we just installed a low-profile toilet not only for better bowel movements but also for the added benefit of deep squatting to get to the seat. And never mind then the added bonus of standing up again from that low position. That is a workout.

It is so odd to me that we have taken basic movement out of our lives to help us be more productive and then we realize that what we had actually done was making us less productive so we created the fitness industry to bring movement back into our lives. There are those who think that they only can move and exercise when they are in a designated workout space, with the right work-out clothes on, at the scheduled time, and then and only then can they work out. This is the totally wrong mind set.

Moving throughout the day is the key. I call this "Creating the Work IN." Adding short duration, simple movement throughout your day allows for this movement addition to be integrated into the landscape of the day. This becomes part of your day as opposed to the typical Work OUT that disrupts the day's flow and perhaps gets put on the back burner as the day's events unfold.

We are all so busy working that we get caught up in the task at hand and we forget to move. Or even worse, our inactive day has drained our energy so that we have no energy to start.

Incorporating the work IN into our day creates and improves energy because ENERGY CREATES MORE ENERGY. And this all starts as soon as we wake up in the morning. When we introduce a physical activity in the morning—right when we wake up—we are oxygenating the blood, generating blood flow to the brain, raising our metabolism, and most of all—opening our thoughts to mindfulness about moving throughout the day.

This mindfulness message is so important for all behavior change. If we want to change a behavior, we need to be mindful of the choices we make. Every action carries with it a subsequent reaction and that can either work for or against wellness. How we eat, how we move throughout the day, who we hang out with, all contribute to the whole picture of wellness.

This work IN can be achieved easily with the following steps:

1. Assess your Work IN day. Write down everything you do on a typical day from the time you wake until the time you go to bed. See template Work-In worksheet below.

2. Highlight the inactivity periods in your day that last longer than one hour and also take note of where you are.

3. Make a list of activities that are possible for a minute or less in the environment that you are in.

4. Commit to one exercise or stretch each morning before getting out of bed.

5. Set a timer, and every 15 minutes of inactivity, GET UP and MOVE.

6. Change up the angle in which your body moves. Use all three planes of movement: a) Sagittal plane—moving front to back, b) Frontal plane—moving side to side, and c) transverse plane—bending, turning, twisting cumulatively throughout the activities chosen. Also choose muscle utilization variety as well. For example, at 9:30, stand and sit 10 times. At 9:45, stand and side bend to each side 5 times each. At 11:00, lunge front to back 5 times on each side.

7. After every meal take a walk and after dinner take a longer walk, jog, or short run.

8. Commit to moving whenever possible. Here is a list of some of my favorites. For 70 "One Minute to Wellness Workouts," just log on to my website and view on onedaytowellness.org. You can do these one-minute workouts anytime anywhere. And there is no excuse as I created these for you for free.

   a. Take the stairs whenever possible—Dahhh but do you actually do this?

   b. Drink lots of water so that you have to get up often to use the restroom.

   c. When you are about to sit, change your mind—sit to stand again—10 times and you have just performed 10 squats.

   d. While waiting in line, squeeze then un-squeeze the glutes muscles or Kegel 10 times. Yes, men have Kegel muscles too. Just squeeze down there and you are doing it right.

   e. While driving, sit up straight and do sitting knee lifts at red lights.

   f. While cooking dinner, turn on dance music instead of the TV and dance while cooking.

   g. Create an environment in your home that stimulates fitness by keeping various pieces of simple fitness equipment in easy access for use. A pair of gliding discs (glidingdiscs.com) in the living room, a stability ball in the TV room, a bender ball (https://benderball.store.savvierfitness.com/) in the kitchen. Also include near the equipment a list of exercises that only take a minute.

h. Create a standup work space. I am typing from one right now. I spend very little time actually sitting at my desk. I stand to do all office work.

i. Schedule Work-IN meetings and events. We like to call these "Walk and Talk Opportunities." Invite all with you to stand and move no matter what the situation—okay not driving, but that goes for most all else.

j. Until you have created the habit of moving throughout the day, keep a movement journal just the same way you keep a food journal. Writing down what you do or don't do keeps you accountable and on track.

Workout Plan #2

I get it that you're busy and that you have no time to exercise. Here is a plan that squeezes the workout seamlessly into your already packed day.

Commit to completing 50 repetitions of five exercises every day of the week. Change every week making sure that the exercises use complementary movement patterns and muscle recruitment.

This week the exercises are 50 each of:

push-ups, sit-ups, tricep dips, squat jumps, and single leg step-ups.

Take a walk or jog after dinner and stretch before bed. Research shows that gentle stretching before bed time can lead to a restful sleep.

Fill in the metabolic profile below and anytime you see you are idle for more than 30 minutes at a time, pick 2-3 of my "One Minute to Wellness" workouts that can be found on onedaytowellness.org or choose any total body exercise to do for a one-minute work-in multiple times a day.

The Work IN Worksheets

This is a sample day for someone who is inactive. How could this person add Work INs?

Time	Activity	Environment	Work In
7-8	Wake, shower, eat breakfast, and drive to work	Home and Car	
8-9	Sit at a desk	Office	
9-10	Sit at a desk	Office	
10-11	Walk to bathroom and back to desk. Sit at desk.	Office	
11-12	Sit at desk	Office	
12-1	Walk to café, sit for lunch, walk back to desk	Outside and Restaurant	
1-2	Sit at desk	Office	
2-3	Sit at desk	Office	
3-4	Sit at desk	Office	
4-5	Sit at desk	Office	
5-6	Drive to gym, take a Tabata Bootcamp class, drive home	Car and Gym	
6-7	Make and eat dinner	Home	
7-8	Watch TV	Home	
8-9	Watch TV and go to bed	Home	

Fill in this activity chart from the time you wake up to the time you go to bed. Notice your inactive times. Add movement during those idle times.

Time	Activity	Environment	Work In
7-8			
8-9			
9-10			
10-11			
11-12			
12-1			
1-2			
2-3			
3-4			
4-5			
5-6			
6-7			
7-8			
8-9			
9-10			

TAKEAWAY TIP

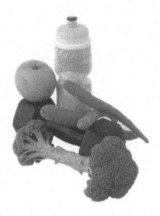

Whether you have an hour a day to work out or no time at all, adding the work-in multiple times a day will lead to health and wellness gains. Work smarter not harder by knowing when to work and when to rest. Intense physical effort requires ample recovery periods so know when to push and when to back off.

1. Mix up your workouts between steady-state and interval HIIT training. incorporating cardio, strength, and stretching
2. Work IN throughout the day functionally for mobility and stability and lifelong capability
3. Stretch at night before bed for a restful sleep

PENIS TIP – BOYS AND BIKE SEATS

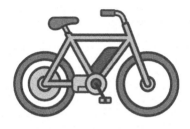

When our boys were young, Bruce and I took every opportunity to get away for a romantic weekend which happened few and far between. With me working full time on the fitness convention circuit and Bruce working a fuller than full 8 A.M.-6 P.M. as a savvy sales exec, those weekends were gold to us. One such romantic getaway took us to Napa, CA, in the heart of the wine country. Our plan was to bike ride all over Napa and then to spend every evening doing everything romantically possible. We awoke the first morning eager to start our adventure. We mounted our bikes and off we went. Turns out that is the last thing that Bruce mounted all weekend.

Six hours in, we had made our way back to our hotel ready for action. No kids, a great day of sightseeing, and mama wants what mamma wants. Well, let's just say nothing was moving—nothing, nada, niltch. Try and try again, but Bruce was numb. Doorknob numb. The bike seat had done him in. Tip—Don't plan a six-hour bike tour with your honey if you want any action whatsoever because it ain't gonna happen.

Tip About the Tip

The perineum does not like prolonged pressure. Anything that places pressure on the pudendal artery can result in penile numbness and impotence.

KITCHEN STAPLES AND SHORTCUTS

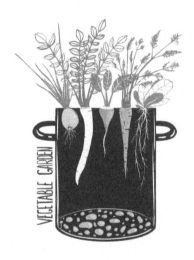

*Whenever you find yourself on the side of
the majority, it's time to pause and reflect.*

— Mark Twain

It is important to set up your kitchen environment for
success. Fall in love with your kitchen. This should be
your favorite room in the house. It is imperative to
stock your kitchen full of not only delicious and nutritious

food but also with what I call Quickies for when you are short on time. I have listed kitchen gadgets that are a must for preparation and storage as well as specific food brands that Bruce and I love. Any brands you see listed can all be purchased online as I don't know where you live and online shopping comes to you. Also, please know that our foundation, One Day to Wellness, is a nonprofit, so we do not accept any royalties from any of the brands listed. These are just our fav's that you may benefit knowing about.

These brands made the cut because most are non-GMO (non-Genetically Modified Organisms), organic, with no added salt, sugar, or oil. They are also the most delicious and nutritionally dense out there. These items are the staples you should have on hand.

Refrigerator and Pantry Essentials

Bread and muffins - Ezekiel -
   https://www.foodforlife.com/about_us/ezekiel-49

Dried beans and popcorn - Rancho Gordo -
   https://www.ranchogordo.com/

Canned or boxed beans - Eden Foods -
   https://www.edenfoods.com/store/beans/beans-
   canned.html

Mustard - Kozliks - https://www.kozliks.com/

Flour and Grains - Bob's Red Mill -
   https://www.bobsredmill.com/

156

Pasta Sauce - Engine 2 - https://plantstrong.com/tomato-basil-pasta-sauce

Canned fire roasted tomatoes - Muir Glen https://www.muirglen.com/products/tomato-sauce/

Hummus Engine 2 - https://plantstrong.com/traditional-hummus

Crackers - Mary's Gone Crackers - https://www.marysgonecrackers.com/

Soy milk - WestSoy organic unsweetened plain soy milk - http://www.westsoymilk.com/

Plant-based yogurt - Forager Cashewmilk yogurt alternative unsweetened https://www.foragerproject.com/all-products/dairy-free-yogurt/

Plant-based burgers - Engine 2 black bean burger - https://plantstrong.com/poblano-black-bean-burger

Balsamic Vinegar - Olivewood - https://www.amazon.com/ACETAIA-CATTANI-Olivewood-Balsamic-8-5/dp/B00BDB0ICU

Nutritional yeast, apple cider vinegar, liquid aminos - Bragg -https://www.bragg.com/

Buckwheat soba pasta - Eden Foods - https://www.edenfoods.com/store/soba-100-buckwheat.html

Oatmeal - Bob's Red Mill - https://www.bobsredmill.com/shop/oats.html

Flax seeds - Bob's Red Mill - https://www.bobsredmill.com/golden-flaxseed.html

Jackfruit canned - The Jackfruit Company - https://thejackfruitcompany.com/

Plant milks - Three Trees - https://www.threetrees.com/

Fruit spreads - Fiorifrutta - https://www.rigonidiasiago-usa.com/fiordifrutta-products/

Nut butter - Artisana - https://artisanaorganics.com/collections/pure-raw-nut-butters

Tempeh - 100% Plant-based protein (tempeh, burgers, smart dogs) - https://lightlife.com/

Chocolate - Theo - https://theochocolate.com/

Alter Eco - chocolate - https://www.alterecofoods.com/

Kitchen Tools

Preparing food is so easy when you have the right tools and they are stored within reach where you are sure to use them. A kitchen tool is only as good as how many times it gets used. Store your most used items on the counter or within easy access.

Always on My Counter:

Coffeemaker—Basic Mr. Coffee 12-cup coffee maker because we drink a lot of coffee and I don't really like the bells and whistles that more expensive coffee makers come with. If you swear by your fancy Italian drip expresso maker—great and go for it. More than a few buttons on anything makes my head spin.

Coffee Tip—How do you like your coffee? Try making your coffee-addition choices the healthiest they can be. How about hemp, or soy, or almond, or cashew, or oat milk? If you like your coffee more on the sweeter side, try date syrup. Date syrup has the most antioxidants compared to other sweeteners. Molasses comes in second. All other sweeteners score fairly low.

Toaster—Oster 4-slot as we eat a lot of toast and we need four slots at all times.

Toast Tip—Choose whole grain bread and top with raw nut butter and fruit. Try using your toaster for more than just toast—try thinly sliced sweet potatoes, organic stone ground corn tortillas, and use to reheat pancakes and thinly sliced muffins.

Hot Water Kettle—Always having the ability to easily heat water for tea or lemon water is a must. You may have the ability to get hot water on demand from your faucet, and this is even better as it frees up counter space. Another option too is to keep a kettle on the stove for easy access.

Warm Beverage Tip—For a warm spicy beverage try mixing hot water with ½ teaspoon dried ginger and cayenne pepper with 1 tablespoon honey and lemon juice.

In the Cabinet:

Food Processor—In our brick and mortar home (that we own but are currently not living there) we have a very expensive Cuisinart that Bruce and I got as a wedding gift almost 40 years ago and it is still going strong. However, it is quite heavy for the RV life so I have opted for the Hamilton Beach food processor which I actually like better. It has suction cups on its base so it doesn't gyrate off the counter during use. It has a food scraper built right in so there is no need to start and stop to take off the lid to scrape the sides of the bowl. And it is cheap—around 40 to 50 bucks.

Food Processor Tip—after reading through the recipes, you may want your food processer to just live on your counter. My chocolate mousse and nut butter recipes alone will have you using it multiple times a week. We also own a small version as well for the smaller jobs. You might want to invest in this as well as sometimes the larger food processor is too large and that might deter you from using any processor at all.

Crock Pot, Rice Cooker, or Instant Pot—We own the Aroma brand rice/soup cooker and it works just fine. We know people who swear by their Instant Pots. Either way, owning one of these is non-negotiable. All you need to do is, literally throw veggies, beans, potatoes, water, spices into this beauty, close the lid, and in a very short period of time you have created a culinary masterpiece. I make at least one soup or stew a week that lasts at least three days. I assure you, you don't need any cooking expertise to whip up an amazing soup or stew. Just follow the recipes in the soups section, and you are sure to impress.

Crock Pot Tip—The inner pot is removable from the cooker itself and you may think to just use that pot as storage of the soup or stew or rice or oatmeal that you have just cooked. Instead of that, transfer the food into a glass storage container. This will allow you to always have the pot available to cook something else. It is too easy to not cook because what you want to use to cook with is otherwise occupied. You also now have your cooked items in a container that can easily be reheated in the microwave.

Heavy-Duty Blender—The Vitamix is the top of the line and I own this, but I really like the Ninja. The blades run all the way up the center of the blender, and the cost is much less. It is also lighter weight and easier to move here and there. But again, we have a Vitamix at home, and it has done the job.

Blender Tip—There are jobs where the blender works better than the food processor and vice versa. For my chocolate mousse recipe, the blender works better when blending the liquid (dates and water to form date paste) but I prefer the food processor for blending the remaining ingredients. So basically, if it is a beverage or more liquid ingredients, go with the blender.

Coffee Grinder—The coffee grinder is not only to grind coffee but also to grind flax seed. If you have downloaded and are following the Daily Dozen food log app that was highlighted in the "Tips to Transition" chapter, you know that flax seeds are a food to be eaten every day. And the best way to eat them as also mentioned earlier is to grind them about every 2-3 days so that they are as fresh as possible. The coffee grinder can also grind certain spices if you happen to purchase whole spice seeds.

Yonana Ice Cream Maker—this is a must if you love ice cream and frozen desserts. As I mentioned earlier, this frozen banana ice cream maker has been our go-to for that "I gotta have a smooth creamy delicious sweet treat right now" without the health detriments of dairy.

Yonana Tip—the Yonana ice cream maker is no good without frozen bananas. Whenever you are at the store look for the spottiest, past their prime bananas you can find. Buy them, bring them home, peel them, and stick them in your freezer. Always have these ready to go at a moment's notice when the urge strikes.

In Your Kitchen Drawers:

Three sharp knives—one large, one serrated, and a paring knife.

Knife Tip—A good sharp knife is your best friend in the kitchen. Get rid of your old dull knives and go buy yourself some really good knives. Wash by hand and not in the dishwasher. Your knives will stay sharper longer.

Our great friend and fellow whole-food plant-based advocate, Jeff Llewellyn, shared this knife tip: "For me another kitchen staple, given 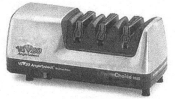 how much chopping we do, is a really good Santoku or Chef's knife; as well as a good knife-sharpener. We have a Chef's Choice 1520 and it takes about a minute to put a really good edge back on a knife. I call dull knives smushers because they just smush a tomato instead of cutting through it!"

Basic Utensils and Accessories:

1. Ladle for soup and stew serving
2. A large non-metal non-stick spoon for stirring
3. A non-metal non-stick spatula
4. A non-metal non-stick whisk for whisking
5. And most importantly these toast tongs—for around seven bucks, these tongs have saved many tortillas and toast when they got stuck at the bottom of the toaster.

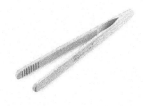

Non-stick Cookware

Because using added oil to cook with is not necessary, preheat the pan and then use any of the following: Wine, balsamic vinegar, water, mustard, vegetable broth, fruit juice. Anything is better than oil. Taste the goodness of the food and not the liquid fat that it is cooked in.

Glass Storage Containers

Because you will be batch-cooking, you will need lots of storage containers that can easily go from fridge to microwave to oven. Glass is always best. It is not a good idea to microwave anything in plastic. According to studies outlined in the article, "Is plastic a threat to your health?" heating food in plastic can leach plastic into the food.

The article states:

> Studies have found that certain chemicals in plastic can leach out of the plastic and into the food and beverages we eat. Some of these chemicals have been linked to health problems such as metabolic disorders (including obesity) and reduced fertility. This leaching can occur even faster and to a greater degree when plastic is exposed to heat. This means you might be getting an even higher dose of potentially harmful chemicals simply by microwaving your leftovers in a plastic container.

The takeaway is, put this book down right now and go buy yourself glass bowls and storage containers.

Parchment Paper and Parchment Muffin Papers

First off, throw away the cooking spray. You don't need it. And it isn't doing your health any favors. Fat is fat whether it comes in a jar, spray, or can. Use parchment paper instead in the oven to:

1. Roast your veggies and your nuts
2. Bake your cookies and sweet potatoes

Use parchment paper muffin papers for cupcakes and muffins.

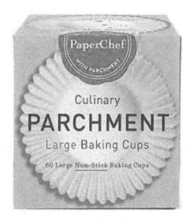

Accessories to Purchase

Purchase these only if you will use them, and you have a ton of storage space. Don't purchase any gadget just because it is the newest latest greatest. Start with the basics and then add more when you have gotten the hang of the simple stuff. Less is better when it comes to the kitchen. This is why, in my recipe section, you see simple ingredients, simple instructions, and simple prep and clean up. The more gadgets the more set up, maintenance, and clean up.

- Air Fryer—bought but rarely use.
- Water Purifier—Use every day so this should probably go into my must haves.
- Waffle Maker—This is great on special occasions.
- Flour Mill—We use this to grain our wheat berries to make bread, but you can easily purchase whole grain flour.
- Bread Maker—This I own and never use as I mix the dough by hand.
- Juicer—We blend our smoothies, but I know people who swear by their juicers.

Shortcuts—Quickies

There are those times when life is crazy and you haven't preplanned, prepared, or prepped a thing. With the following shortcuts in your back pocket, you will never have to resort to fast fake food ever again.

1. Frozen is fine. Try to buy organic as often as possible. Stock your freezer with frozen berries for smoothies or oatmeal for breakfast. Frozen precut veggies are so easy to toss into soups and stews. Frozen edamame (after they are reheated) make for a wonderful snack.
2. Canned is fine. Just read the label to make sure you are choosing salt, sugar, and oil free. Canned

beans can be used for soups, stews, and hummus, or on a salad. Diced or chopped tomatoes are a shortcut for stir fry, soups, and stews as well. Apple sauce is a great substitute for oil or butter in baking. Canned veggies and fruit are also an a-okay—just go for the one-ingredient varieties.

3. Have a loaf of pre-sliced whole grain bread and/or some English muffins in the freezer for easy toasted PBJ's. Or use store-bought hummus or avocados for toast with the most.

4. If you have a Whole Foods nearby, check out the Engine 2 brand. All items are salt, sugar, and oil free from their pasta sauce to their hummus to their plant-based burgers. Many of the items are prepared and ready to eat while others only need reheating.

5. If you are so short on time that eating in is not an option at all, then here are your best bets for eating out.

a. Grocery Store—The salad bar is a great choice as you have control of what items you choose. Just watch oil dressings. Instead, choose balsamic vinegar, Bragg Liquid Aminos, lemon squeeze, and nutritional yeast.

b. Steak or Sea Food Restaurant—At a steak res-taurant choose a baked potato with steamed veggies. If you are going to order seafood, go for smaller fish on the food chain that are wild-caught with minimal sauce.

   c. Mexican—Mexican is easy. Ask for the sides as your main course. Pico de gallo or salsa, avocado, rice and beans, and steamed corn tortillas. And do your best to skip the chips.

   d. Asian—There are rice and steamed veggies, veggies rolls, and wok dishes without added oil. Ask for water to be used in the wok instead of oil.

   e. Italian—Steamed veggies with a side of pasta with marinara. If you ask for pasta with veggies, you will end up with a plate of pasta with one sprig of broccoli. Be very specific and ask for exactly what you want.

   f. Fast Food—Drive on by as there are better options right down the street. If fast food is your only option, opt for any veggies that are available, and ketchup and French fries don't count.

TAKE AWAY TIPS

When your kitchen is ready for action, so are you. Take the time to set up your kitchen for success and you will reap the rewards of healthy eating at every meal.

1. Spend money on kitchen tools that will save you tons in the long run. Invest in non-stick cookware and appliances that will last a lifetime and will be used every day.
2. Display daily-used items on the counter and have them within easy access so that there will be no excuse for not cooking at home.
3. Stock your kitchen full of all the staples you need and have on hand grab-and-go snacks so that eating healthy is not only delicious, it is easy and well thought out.

PENIS TIP –
BORN WITH ONE AND DIE WITH ONE

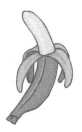

I never wanted to know the sex of any of our sons before they were born. Their names didn't even need to change depending on the sex as all have unisex names. It was our third son, however, who showed himself loud and clear while still in utero. During one of our OB visits, he let all hang out during that particular ultrasound. No mistaking what that was. Boy was that boy hung. Well, it turns out that erections actually are a thing in the womb. I wouldn't have believed it unless I saw it.

Even more crazy is the death erection or also coined the angel lust or terminal erection. This erection pops up after the man has died. Okay, to be clear, this usually only happens under morbid circumstances—hanging, gunshot to the head, or poisoning. Rare, yes, but true.

PLANT POWERED RECIPES
FOR REAL MEN

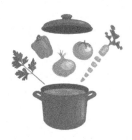

World Peace begins in the kitchen.

— Anonymous

Google "vegan no oil *best for sexual performance recipes*" and what will pop up is a plethora of enticing options for every occasion. This chapter highlights my favorites, sure to please even the most die-hard carnivore. These recipes are compiled within meal themes—breakfast, lunch/dinner, and dessert/snack—but all are interchangeable and can be eaten at any time of day or eve depending on your preference. I have not only chosen these based on their health benefits, but also for their tastiness and ease of preparation. These recipes are also created to substitute for your current staples like burgers, pizza, lasagna, cookies, muffins, and French toast.

Make sure you read the chapter, "Kitchen Staples and Shortcuts" to help with preparation. If you don't like to cook, don't fear as these recipes are so simple and easy that anyone can make them. As stated throughout this book, include your significant other in all this as cooking together is an aphrodisiac to the tenth degree. Trust me. I think all three of our boys were conceived right there in the kitchen.

Breakfast
1. Groats
2. Steel Cut Oatmeal
3. Overnight Oats
4. Pumpkin Muesli Muffins
5. Buckwheat Pancakes
6. Wilted Greens
7. Super Power Shake
8. Flax French Toast
9. Tofu Scramble

Lunch /Dinner
1. Instant Pot or Pot-on-the-Stove-Cooker Soup Variations
   a. Split Pea Soup
   b. Bean and Veggie Soup
   c. Sweet Potato and Tomato Soup
   d. Lentil and Potato Soup from my friend Riley Shaia

e. Black Lentil and Fire Roasted Tomato Soup

f. Chick Pea and Butternut Squash Soup

g. Quick-and-Easy Mighty Bean Chili

2. Better-than-Burger Burgers

    a. Black Bean Burger with Quinoa

    b. Oatmeal Black Bean Burger

    c. Beet Burger

3. Toast with the Most

    a. Whole Wheat Bread

    b. Avocado Toast (Simple Recipe)

    c. Homemade Nut Butter

    d. Hummus, Tomato, and Greens Toast

4. Italian Stallion Dishes

    a. Soy Curls with Pesto

    b. Spaghetti Squash Lasagna

    c. Shortcut Lasagna

    d. Plant Powered Pizza

5. Savory Sides

    a. Cauliflower Mash

    b. Vegetable Lentil Salad

    c. Stuffed Pesto Mushrooms

    d. Vegetable Rice Stuffed Peppers

    e. Cauli-Power Vegetable Risotto

6. Bruce's Best

    a. Tempeh Mushroom Stir Fry

    b. Jackfruit BBQ

    c. What every salad shouldn't go without - Bruce's Killer Salad Dressing

    d. Bruce's Killer Super Picker-Upper Snack

Dessert / Snack

1. Mindy's Famous Balls (Date and Nut Ball Variations)
2. Roasted Chestnuts
3. Chocolate Mousse
4. Black Bean Brownies
5. Chickpea Cookie Dough
6. Oatmeal Banana Cookies
7. Chocolate Fudge Pudding
8. Pecan Bars
9. Chia Pudding

BREAKFAST

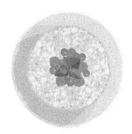

Groats

What are Groats? Groats are intact grains that contain their germ and endosperm. Groats are whole grains that are closest to the source of where they came from. Groats are full of soluble fiber and are the least processed of all the grains. Groats keep you fuller longer than more processed grains. Oat groats are intact grain while steel cut oats have been cut 2-3 times and old-fashioned oats have been crushed. When Bruce and I first transitioned from eating the traditional standard America diet breakfast of eggs, bacon, and white bagels with cream cheese, we chose old fashioned oatmeal as our transition. As our nutritional education expanded, we traded in the old-fashioned oatmeal for steel cut oatmeal. Now that we know how much more nutritious grains in their purest form are, we are all in with the groats.

The beauty of where you are right now is that you can jump right on the groats train. You don't have to cipher through the journey of discovery. We have already done that for you. All you need to do is sit back and reap the benefits of our travels to where we are now. When Bruce and I started on this whole food, plant-based journey, we knew very little about the implementation piece. Through trial-and-error and fail-and-succeed we are where we are today. You are in the perfect place as there are so many like us who have learned the hard way and paved the way for all of you new, whole food, plant-based pioneers.

If you want to take baby steps, here is both a tried-and-true steel cut and overnight oat recipe. When you are ready to groat it up, go either to the bulk section of your grocery store or if your grocery store doesn't have a dried bulk section, move—no, just kidding. You can purchase all groats on the internet at Amazon or Bob's Red Mill.

Groats to try:

Oat
Buckwheat
Farrow
Kamut—our favorite
Millet
Quinoa
Amaranth
Barley

To shorten the cooking time, soak overnight in water. The next morning, drain the soaking water and replace with fresh water that covers the groats and allow just short of an inch more water at the top. Cook on medium heat on the stove for 10-30 minutes depending on the grain chosen. The smaller the groats, the quicker they cook. Always batch cook. This means make enough for at least three meals.

Steel Cut Oatmeal

Steel cut oatmeal is an excellent choice for any time of day. Top with flax seed, nuts, and berries, and you have a complete meal.

4 cups water
2 cups steel cut oatmeal

Instructions:

1. Add ingredients together in pot on stove top or in an Instant Pot.
2. Cook on stove (according to package time).
3. Top with maple syrup, date syrup, walnuts, almonds, cashews, ground flax seed, berries of all types (fresh or frozen), motherless milk (soy, hemp, almond), oat, seeds, almond or peanut butter, currents and raisins, chopped apples, bananas, peaches—any fruit and all fruit.
4. Make enough for at least three meals. Store in premeasured packs either in fridge or freezer for easy reheating in microwave or stove top.

Overnight Oats

Uncooked rolled oats use the most processed oat grain—the old-fashioned oat. This oat processing cuts, then crushes the oat groats into a flat flake. This allows the oat to have less cooking time and can be used in baking and uncooked rolled oats as the oats don't need to be cooked to be easily digested.

2 cups overnight oats
2 cups plant milk—I like oat milk because
    it is the sweetest of the plant milks.
¼ cup raisins or currents or both
1 teaspoon cinnamon
1 tablespoon ground flax seeds
1 tablespoon chia seeds (optional)
Depending on your taste also add
¼ cup cacao powder
1 cut up banana
or
1 cup fresh berries—blueberries, strawberries,
    or blackberries
or
1 cup fruit—apples, peaches, pears
or
½ cup nut butter

Instructions:

1. Add ingredients together.
2. Store in refrigerator overnight.
3. Enjoy alone or with added motherless milk or heated up.

Pumpkin Muesli Muffins

These muffins are moist and filling, and are good for on the go or as a side to your breakfast wilted greens. Drizzle Forager cashew unsweetened yogurt (or another unsweetened plant-based yogurt) and berries on top for a fabulous dessert. Or dip into my chocolate pudding—yum.

1 cup spelt flour

1 cup almond flour

½ cup muesli

2 teaspoons baking soda

2 teaspoons baking powder

1 teaspoon cinnamon

¼ teaspoon nutmeg

6 tablespoons date sugar

1 tablespoon ground flax seed

1¼ cup oat milk

1 cup pumpkin

1 tablespoon lemon juice

1½ tablespoons vanilla

Instructions:

1. Preheat oven to 350 F.
2. Mix together all dry ingredients.
3. Add wet ingredients to dry ingredients and mix completely.
4. Line muffin tin with parchment paper muffin cups.
5. Bake in preheated 350 F oven for 20-30 minutes or until done.

Buckwheat Pancakes

Buckwheat flour is packed with antioxidants and minerals and is gluten-free if that is important to you. Make enough for at least three days so that you can reheat in the toaster as a snack or use instead of bread for a PBJ. They also are great frozen and reheated days later.

½ cup each buckwheat and another flour (almond, spelt, whole wheat—really any is fine just as long as it is whole grain)
1 cup oat milk
1 teaspoon vanilla
1 teaspoon cinnamon
½ teaspoon baking powder
2 tablespoon ground flax seed

Instructions:

1. Mix all ingredients together with a whisk until blended.
2. Preheat a non-stick fry pan (this is crucial as this will determine if the first batch is a winner or a loser).
3. Cook on preheated non-stick fry pan until done.
4. Top with maple syrup, berries, nut butter, date syrup, cashew yogurt, or have just all by themselves.

Wilted Greens

Cruciferous veggies should be the stable of your diet every day, and what better time to get them then the morning at breakfast? Breakfast is, so many times, a wasted opportunity to pack in nutrition. Breakfast literally means breaking the fast—eating after not eating—and how you fuel yourself will set the stage for the rest of the day. There is a mindset that if the day starts with eating crap, then the day is written off and the rest of the day's meals are made up of crap. So, what happens when you eat crap? You feel like crap—and most likely you don't crap. So that crap is stuck inside of you for literally days. YUCK. Start the day off right, and the rest of the day may just proceed in the same way—right? Wilted Greens are THE right way to start the day. With enough fiber, protein, and antioxidants to fuel the entire day, how could the rest of the day go anywhere but right?

2-4 cloves of garlic diced

1 large onion diced

4 cups of power greens—spinach, kale, collards, chard

¼ teaspoon all-purpose seasoning—no salt

¼ teaspoon ground pepper

¼ cup white wine

2 tablespoons mustard

3 tablespoons balsamic vinegar

Instructions:

1. Preheat non-stick fry pan on stove.
2. Put the wine, mustard, and vinegar in the pan wine.
3. Add garlic and onion to the liquid; let cook for 4-6 minutes.
4. Add seasonings.

5. Add greens until all have wilted but not cooked all the way to mush
6. Serve on toast with salsa, hot sauce, avocado, spices

Super Power Shake

Short on time? Then the power shake is the way to go. This power shake allows you to get in all your vitamins and minerals, fiber, and protein in one easy-to-prepare and easy-to-swallow liquid beverage. Change up the taste by switching fruits, veggies, juices, and motherless milks. For a creamier texture, add nut butter or banana or plant milks. For a lighter brighter taste, go for berries, juice, or water.

Thick and Creamy Power Shake

1 banana
1 cup oat or other plant milk
1-2 tablespoons nut butter
2 tablespoons cacao powder
1 teaspoon ground flax seed
½ cup pitted dates
½ cup raw spinach
1 cup ice

Instructions:

Mix all in a high-powered blender until blended.

Fruity and Fresh Power Shake

1 cup spinach
1 cup frozen berries

1 orange peeled
½ cup pomegranate juice
½ cup water or more if needed
1 cup ice

Instructions:

1. Mix all in a high-powered blender until blended.
2. Drink up

Flax French Toast

Who doesn't love French toast? As an addition to your breakfast rotation of groats and wilted greens, French toast makes for an amazing weekend splurge without the health downside, only upside with these ingredients

5-6 Slices whole grain thick, hearty bread
2 tablespoons ground chia or flax seeds
1 tablespoon maple syrup
1 cup unsweetened plant milk
1 tablespoon ground cinnamon
1 tablespoon vanilla extract

Instructions:

1. Preheat a non-stick fry pan on the stove at medium heat.
2. Mix all ingredients except bread together in a large bowl and let sit for 10 minutes.
3. Dip both sides of bread into mixture and toast on pan, turning from side to side until done.
4. Top with maple syrup, fruit, nut butter, plant yogurt, dried fruit, cinnamon, or date sugar, and enjoy.

Tofu Scramble

Forget everything you have heard about eggs—eggs are not a health food. Studies show that even eating just two eggs a week can increase your risk of diabetes and heart disease. In March 2019, researchers from four universities who had been following collectively 29,615 U.S. adults for an average of 17.5 years published the results of the research in *JAMA* (The Journal of the American Medical Association). They found that those participants who ate an average of two eggs per day had a 27% increased risk of developing heart disease.

And why even eat eggs, when this tofu scramble is so much tastier and better for you? Mix in all your favorite veggies, top with salsa and avocado, and serve on whole grain toast, and you will never miss the egg.

1 package organic tofu firm
1 large onion minced
3-4 garlic cloves minced
Your favorite chopped veggies—bok choy, collards, Kale, mushrooms, bell peppers
Spices—Season to taste with pepper, all-purpose no-salt seasoning, Bragg Liquid Aminos, vinegar, dill

Instructions:

1. Preheat a skillet on stove on medium heat.
2. Sauté onion and garlic in veggie broth or white wine or both
3. Add chopped veggies, tofu, and seasonings to the pan

4. Cook stirring often, only until all veggies are wilted
5. Serve on toasted whole grain bread
6. Top with salsa, avocado, hot sauce, vinegar

LUNCH / DINNER

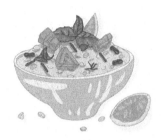

A quick note—I have under-seasoned everything on purpose. You want to under-season so that you have somewhere to go when tasting after the dish is fully cooked. If you use too many spices right off the bat, there is no going back, and you are stuck with overly seasoned food. As you are transitioning to eating more whole natural foods, your taste buds will start to become sensitive again to how the real food tastes. You will discover that you will start to use less and less salt, sugar, and oil. Trust me and follow my directions and then taste the finished dish. If then, and only then, you feel that you need a little more of this or that, add it to taste—and not to habit.

Instant Pot or Pot-on-the-Stove-Cooker Soup Variations

Split Pea Soup
Bean and Veggie Soup
Sweet Potato Tomato Soup
Lentil and Potato Soup
Black Lentil and Fire Roasted Tomato Soup
Chick Pea and Butternut Squash Stew
Quick and Easy Mighty Bean Chili

Split Pea Soup

I buy split peas in the 5 lb. bag on Amazon because I find myself always running out. Split peas are creamy, filling, and are tasty both al dente and cooked through and through.

This soup will be your favorite on those cold winter eves.

6 cups water or no sodium vegetable broth
½ cup white wine
2 cups uncooked green split peas rinsed
1 large onion, chopped
1 cup chopped carrots
1 cup celery with leaves, chopped
2 garlic cloves, minced
1 teaspoon no-salt all-purpose seasoning
½ teaspoon dried basil
2-3 dried bay leaves
½ teaspoon ground cumin
¾ teaspoon pepper

Instructions:

Throw everything in an Instant Pot or on the stove pot and cook between 45 minutes to 1 hour. For a smooth soup blend or for a chunky soup, eat as is.

Bean and Veggie Soup

This soup is a meal—no doubt about it. Serve with warm toasted bread and you are good to go. Play around with the veggies you add because there is no wrong way to go here.

2 cups dried soaked beans—black beans, white Northern beans, kidney beans, pinto beans, peas— your choice. If you are short on time, used no salt canned beans.

6 cups water or veggie broth

1 large onion chopped

2-4 garlic cloves chopped

3-4 tomatoes chopped and 1 can chopped tomatoes

Your choice of veggies—carrots, celery, bok choy, peas, corn, fennel

1 teaspoon each cumin, parsley, all-purpose seasoning, paprika, pepper

Instructions:

1. In an Instant Pot or on the stove, add all ingredients together. As beans take longer than lentils or canned beans, allow for more cooking time. Again, if short on time, use canned beans.
2. Cook until done.
3. Season to taste.

Sweet Potato and Tomato Soup

What makes this such an amazing stick-to-your-ribs soup is the sweet potato addition. Sweet potatoes add such a unique texture and flavor and fill you up fast.

2 cans diced tomatoes
2 large sweet potatoes cubed
1 large onion chopped
1 bulb garlic minced
5-6 large carrots chopped
2 cups button or cremini mushrooms chopped
6-8 stalks of celery chopped
4 cups water or no sodium vegetable broth
¼ cup white wine (or water)
1 tablespoon all-purpose seasoning
1 bay leaf
1 teaspoon thyme
1 teaspoon marjoram
1 tablespoon paprika
2 teaspoon pepper

Instructions:

1. In an Instant Pot or slow cooker, combine all ingredients and cook for 30 minutes to an hour, checking every 10 minutes.
2. Season with only enough salt and additional spices as needed.

Lentil and Potato Soup from my friend Riley Shaia

My friend Riley is one of our One Day to Wellness trainers, but more than that, she is an amazing cook. I travel to her house all the way across the country just to be invited for dinner. So, when I asked her to contribute to my recipe section, I was over joyed when she submitted this one—creamy and dreamy—that's all I'll say.

1 tablespoon water or vegetable broth
1 small onion, minced
1 clove garlic, minced
1 medium potato peeled and cubed
1 small sweet potato or butternut squash, peeled and
    cubed (frozen will also work)
2 medium carrots, cubed
2-3 stalks of celery, diced
2 medium zucchini or squash, diced or cut
1 cup lentils (can be a blend of different types)
5 cups water
1 bay leaf
1 teaspoon thyme
1 teaspoon marjoram
1 teaspoon smoked paprika
1 teaspoon dried rosemary
¼ cup nutritional yeast
salt and pepper to taste

Instructions:

Instant Pot:

1. Turn the Instant Pot on the sauté function and sauté onion in water or vegetable broth until onion is translucent. Add garlic and sauté a few minutes more.

2. Turn off the sauté function and add rest of ingredients except nutritional yeast and salt. Put the lid on, press manual button for 10 minutes.

3. Once finished, allow pressure to come down naturally.

4. Stir in nutritional yeast and salt and pepper to taste.

Black Lentil and Fire Roasted Tomato Soup

What makes this soup a standout is the addition of the fire-roasted tomatoes. I actually didn't have regular canned tomatoes one night and only had fire roasted and threw them in. Wow. What a creative creation.

2 cans no sodium fire roasted diced tomatoes
6 cups water or vegetable broth
¼ cup white wine (optional—maybe for you but not for me)
1 leek chopped
1 fennel chopped
4 large carrots chopped
6 celery stalks with leaves chopped
1 large onion chopped
5 cloves of garlic minced
½ teaspoon Paprika
½ teaspoon cumin
1 tablespoon all-purpose non salt seasoning
1 teaspoon pepper and then more to taste if needed
1 teaspoon Bragg Liquid Aminos
2 cups uncooked black lentils rinsed

Instructions:

1. Combine all ingredients except lentils and cook on soup setting for 10 minutes.
2. Add lentils and cook until done—depending on cooker, around 20-40 minutes.
3. Serve with hot sauce or sriracha if you like it spicy or with nutritional yeast if you like it cheesy and mild. We love to toast organic stone-ground tortillas in the toaster and crumble on top. And sometimes we even mix in brown rice.

Chick Pea and Butternut Squash Soup

This is another contribution from my culinary genius friend Riley. Yum and yum again.

1 medium butternut squash, cut into cubes

2 tablespoons water or no sodium vegetable broth

1 tablespoon black pepper

1 large onion, chopped

1 bulb garlic—about 8-10 cloves finely chopped

½ cup finely chopped parsley

1 tablespoon no-salt all-purpose seasoning

1½ teaspoons ground cumin

1 teaspoon paprika

1 teaspoon cumin

1 teaspoon coriander

1 bay leaf

½ teaspoon cayenne pepper

3 medium carrots, chopped

2½ cups cooked chickpeas (either from dry beans
    or from two 15-oz. cans)
1 can crushed tomatoes (28 oz.)
½ cup flat-leaf parsley leaves, roughly chopped

Instructions:

1. Preheat oven to 375 degrees. Place squash pieces on a baking sheet lined with parchment paper. Sprinkle with a small amount of all-purpose seasoning and pepper. Toss well and roast until golden brown, 45 to 50 minutes.

2. In a large pan, warm 2 tablespoons of water or broth over medium-high heat. Add onions. Cook for 3 to 4 minutes. Stir in garlic and cook for 3 minutes. Stir in all spices and parsley and cook for 1 minute. Add carrots and 1 cup water and chickpea water from the can to the pan. Bring to a boil over high heat. Reduce heat to low and simmer, covered, until carrots are tender, 10 to 12 minutes.

3. Add tomatoes and chickpeas. Raise heat to medium-high and simmer for 10 minutes. Stir in all remaining ingredients and let simmer until tasty.

Quick-and-Easy Mighty Bean Chili

This chili is so easy, so delicious, and so filling. Use soaked or canned beans and if you like it hot, get ready to unleash the spicy peppers. Remember what you read back in the Stand Outs section—get ready for more than just a great meal.

1 large onion chopped

1 bulb garlic (about 8-10 cloves) finely chopped

1 bell pepper

1 cup sliced mushrooms

1 can EACH no-salt black beans, white northern
    beans, kidney beans drained

1 can corn

1 28-oz. can diced tomatoes or 2 cups fresh tomatoes

1 cup tomato sauce

½ to 1 cup water as needed

1 tablespoon chili powder

4-6 finely chopped jalapeno peppers

1½ teaspoons ground cumin

1 teaspoon pepper

1 teaspoon oregano

1 bay leaf

1 teaspoon cayenne pepper

Instructions:

1. Preheat pan and sauté onion garlic
2. Add bell pepper and cook—just about 2-3 minutes
3. Transfer to pot and add remaining ingredients and cook on medium heat or in an Instant Pot for 20-30 minutes, checking every 10 minutes.

Better-than-Burger Burgers

Black Bean Burger with Quinoa

Oatmeal Black Bean Burger

Beet Burger

195

What would a plant powered penis book be without burger recipes? Burgers and boys go together like peas and carrots. Only I would like the burger to be actually made of peas and carrots. So here you go—my favorite burger alternatives, all without oil or animal products! Go ahead, buy the bun, cook these up, and eat just like you would a traditional burger. You won't miss the meat and neither will your arteries and veins.

Black Bean Burger with Quinoa

Black beans and quinoa together! Shut the front door! What could be better? A complete protein source through and through, and so good for you.

½ cup uncooked quinoa

1 chopped onion

6 chopped mushrooms sautéed in a small amount of white wine or water or veg broth

3 garlic cloves minced

1½ cups cooked black beans

3 tablespoons ground flax seed

2 tablespoons hot chili flakes

Pepper to taste

Instructions:

1. Preheat oven to 350 F.
2. Cook quinoa for 10 minutes in 1½ cups water.
3. Cook onion, mushrooms, and garlic with small amount of white wine or water or veg broth in sauce pan for 3-5 minutes.

4. Mix in ½ beans and ½ quinoa—cook for 5 minutes.
5. Process this in food processor.
6. Then add all remaining ingredients and shape into patties.
7. Cook at 350 F for 20-30 minutes.

Oatmeal Black Bean Burger

This burger is the spicier cousin to the one above. I love the variation of the oatmeal as well as the texture and taste which are quite different and flavorful. Top with all your traditional go-to's except any oily goo.

1⅓ cups old fashioned oats
2 cups black beans
¾ cup salsa or pico de gallo
1 tablespoon soy sauce
1½ teaspoon chili powder
½ teaspoon garlic powder
Pepper to taste
½ cup cooked corn

Instructions:

Preheat oven at 375 F

1. Mix together all ingredients except corn in a food processor and blend.
2. Add corn and mix by hand.
3. Form patties and place on parchment covered cookie sheet.
4. Cook at 375 F for 20-30 minutes.

Beet Burger

As you learned in the chapter, "The Power of Plants," Beets help unleash nitric oxide so that your blood can flow freely. Beets also enhance athletic performance, so eat this for lunch and schedule a 10K run for an hour later and you may see a personal best time.

4 cups peeled and shredded beets
1 15-oz. can cooked chickpeas drained
1 cup brown rice cooked
1 tablespoon balsamic vinegar
2 cloves garlic minced
1 teaspoon onion powder
1 teaspoon Bragg Liquid Aminos
Pepper to taste

Instructions:

1. Toss all into a food processor and blend together until the mixture forms a paste.
2. Form into patties and then let them hang out in fridge while the stove pan is preheating.
3. Heat on stove top on preheated non-stick pan until both sides are firm and crispy.
4. Serve on whole grain bun with your favorite toppings.

Toast with the Most

Whole wheat bread
Avocado toast
Homemade nut butter
Oil-free hummus

Whole Wheat Bread Recipe

Only 3-4 ingredients in this delicious nutritious bread. This bread is dense and perfect when used with your avocado and hummus toast.

4 cups whole wheat flour
2 cups warm water
1 pack quick-rise yeast
1 tablespoon maple sugar (optional)

Instructions:

1. Preheat oven to 400 F.
2. Mix together all ingredients together until you have a dense dough.
3. Pour into two parchment paper lined loaf pans.
4. Let rise 1-2 hours.
5. Bake 40 minutes.

Avocado Toast (Simple Recipe)

Who doesn't love avocado toast? Start simple with just mashed avocado, lemon, and pepper. As you get more creative, add garlic, mustard, vinegars, nuts, seeds, sauer-kraut, Bragg Liquid Aminos, whatever you like—but be adventurous.

1 avocado
1-2 garlic cloves minced
½ lemon juice
Pepper to taste
Add to taste but optional
Apple cider vinegar

Balsamic vinegar
Mustard—We love sweet and smokey Kozliks brand
Rice wine vinegar

Instructions:

1. Toast bread and top with avocado mixture.
2. Eat as is or top with arugula, tomatoes, toasted seeds, kimchi or sauerkraut, whatever you love.

Homemade Nut Butter

As mentioned earlier when buying nuts, raw is best, then dry roasted—but steer clear of roasted nuts as most likely there was oil added to the roasting process. If you are a nut-butter lover, you know that for the good stuff you are paying a pretty penny. This is one of the reasons I started making my own. The other reason is that, with homemade nut butter, you can play with your nuts—the sky is the limit—walnuts, cashews, almonds, peanuts, pistachios. Be adventurous and try your nuts in combination to see what tastes best to you.

Any nuts of choice—here are a few examples

1 cup each walnuts, cashews, almonds
1 cup each walnuts, peanuts, almonds
1 cup each cashews, almonds, ½ cup flax seed
1 cup each almonds, walnuts, ½ cup flax seed

Instructions:

1. You must roast nuts before you process them in a food processor. Preheat the oven to roast setting or to 375 F.

2. Line a baking sheet with parchment paper and place all nuts on paper single layer.
3. Roast for 10-20 minutes, turning nuts about every 5 minutes.
4. The nuts are done when they have slightly tanned and are crispy.
5. Process all in food processor until creamy.

Oil Free Hummus

2-3 cups cooked garbanzo beans (these can be canned or cooked)

Other Beans to Try
White Northern
Black
Pinto
Black-eyed peas

1-2 garlic cloves minced
½ lemon squeezed
Pepper
Add to taste
Bragg Liquid Aminos
Tahini
Apple cider vinegar
Mustard
Balsamic vinegar
Rice wine vinegar
Maple syrup
Sriracha

Instructions:

1. Mix together beans, garlic, lemon, and pepper in food processor.
2. Taste and add additional spice to flavor.
3. Use hummus for any and all spreads and dips.

Italian Stallion Dishes

Soy Curls with Pesto (oil-free/cheese-free pesto)
Spaghetti Squash Lasagna
Shortcut Lasagna
Plant Powered Pizza

Soy Curls with Pesto

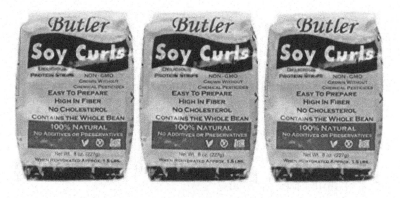

I can only find soy curls on Amazon. Comes in a 3 pack and each pack serves 8-10 people. I usually cook ½ pack at a time as this is one recipe I don't batch cook. I like the taste of these right off the stove smothered in my perfect pesto sauce.

½ to 1 full package soy curls

Water to pre soak

Veggie broth, wine, water to sauté in

Spices of your choice if you are eating these on their own. For the pesto dish, no spice is needed

Instructions:

1. Soak for 10 minutes in water.
2. Drain off the water.
3. Sauté in preheated non-stick frying pan with just enough liquid to sauté in.
4. Add any spices you would like to make the curls taste like what you want them to taste like.
5. Add pesto and share with the neighborhood. They will all convert to leaning more to the green.

OIL FREE / CHEESE FREE PESTO

1 large pack fresh basil—at least 1 cup

1-3 cloves garlic

¼ to ½ cup pine nuts

Juice from one lemon

¼ teaspoon Bragg Liquid Aminos

½ to ¾ cup nutritional yeast

¼ cup tofu or avocado (optional)

Instructions:

1. Add all ingredients into a food processor.
2. Blend together and taste.
3. Add whatever it needs based on your taste (Braggs for salty, nutritional yeast for cheesy, lemon for lemony).

Spaghetti Squash Lasagna

When our friend Riley gave us this recipe to try, I sent Bruce off to the store to pick up all the ingredients. He called me from the store saying that he couldn't find any spaghetti made out of squash. My husband is an amazing chef, but he was unfamiliar with this veggie. Spaghetti squash is actually squash that, when cooked, shreds and has the consistency of spaghetti. Here is a pic of spaghetti squash so you don't have to call anyone from the grocery store.

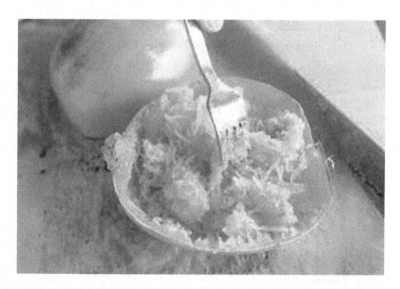

Ingredients:

2 medium spaghetti squash roasted for 1 hour at 350
    degrees
Marinara sauce of your choosing—1-2 jars worth

CHEESY CASHEW SAUCE

1½ cups cashews (soaked overnight)
⅓ cup nutritional yeast
¼ cup + 1 tablespoon lemon juice
1 teaspoon garlic powder
1 teaspoon onion powder
⅔ cup water (more if needed)
1 tsp. salt

Instructions:

1. Blend in high-speed blender until smooth and creamy, adding additional water as needed.
2. Add more salt and lemon juice to taste.

ALMOND PARMESAN CHEESE

½ cup blanched almonds
⅛ cup nutritional yeast
¼ tsp. salt
1 teaspoon garlic powder
1 teaspoon onion powder

Instructions:

Blend in a high -speed blender until mixed.

1. Place a thin layer of marinara on the bottom of a 9 x 13-inch baking dish.
2. Spoon a layer of spaghetti squash, marinara, then "cheese" sauce. Repeat the layers ending with marinara.

3. Sprinkle almond parmesan and fresh basil on top and bake uncovered for 35-45 minutes until heated through.

Shortcut Lasagna

Bruce and I teach a course called Cooking and Coaching. This is an amazing day of cooking a huge assortment of dishes for breakfast, lunch, dinner, and desserts. By the end of the day, when all the dinner items are being prepared, I demonstrate to the group how to make shortcut alternatives to tried-and-true favorites. I came up with this down and dirty lasagna recipe that is just as good as its friend above but takes only minutes to make and cook

Lasagna Noodles—choose the lasagna noodle that you like the best—whole wheat, buckwheat, quinoa, edamame, spelt, or any whole grain pasta.

CASHEW CREAM

1½ cups cashews soaked
⅓ cup nutritional yeast
¼ cup and 1 tablespoon lemon juice
1 teaspoon garlic powder
1 teaspoon onion powder
1 teaspoon salt

Instructions:

Mix together in food processor.

TOMATO SAUCE

1 large jar oil-free tomato sauce—We use Engine 2 company

1 small can tomato paste

1 cup grated carrots

¼ cup chopped basil

6 teaspoons garlic chopped

1 teaspoon thyme

2 teaspoons parsley

2 teaspoons oregano

Instructions:

Heat on stove.

Instructions—Lasagna creation:

Alternate layering whole grain cooked lasagna noodles with cashew cream and tomato sauce. Cook in preheated 350 F oven for 30-40 minutes.

Plant Powered Pizza

If you have a family, schedule pizza night once a week. Take everyone to the grocery store and assign each person a certain number of veggies to choose to use as the topping. Make pizza night special by everyone purchasing and participating in the preparation turning pizza night into a family tradition.

PIZZA DOUGH

1 cup warm water
1 pack yeast
1 tablespoon date sugar or maple syrup
2¾ white whole wheat flour
½ teaspoon salt

TOPPINGS

Pizza or pasta sauce—oil free. If choosing pasta sauce, add a small can of tomato paste to thicken.

Any and all veggies—some you may want to add after cooking as their water content is higher and they may make the pizza too moist.

Nutritional yeast

Hot sauce or hot chili flakes

Instructions:

1. In a large bowl, add the warm water to the flour and yeast.
2. Mix in the sugar or syrup and salt.
3. Mix until dough is firm.
4. Let rise for 1-2 hours.
5. Preheat oven to 425 F.
6. Line a pizza pan with parchment paper.
7. Form dough into pizza shape on pan.
8. Top with canned Engine 2 or another no-oil pizza sauce

9. Add all veggies—peppers, mushrooms, tomatoes, garlic, onion, arugula—any really.
10. Top with nutritional yeast.
11. Cook at 425 F for 8-10 minutes—check center to see if it is done as cooking time varies due to the amount of sauce and veggies you use.

Savory Sides

Cauliflower Mash
Vegetable Lentil Salad
Stuffed Pesto Mushrooms
Vegetable Rice Stuffed Peppers
Cauli-Power Vegetable Risotto

Cauliflower Mash

Cauliflower mash is so easy to prepare and adds the perfect side dish to just about anything. Buy pre-shredded cauliflower, and it almost makes itself. I have no problem at all with mashed potatoes, but this is a savory alternative without added oil or butter.

1 medium cauliflower or 2 cups prepackaged
    shredded cauliflower
2 cloves garlic minced
2 tablespoons nutritional yeast
1 teaspoon all-purpose seasoning salt-free
Pepper and a tiny bit of salt to taste
¼ cup unsweetened motherless milk

Instructions:

1. Steam cauliflower in steamer until soft.
2. At the same time roast garlic on stove in preheated non-stick frying pan.
3. Add both and all other ingredients to food processor.
4. Blend until creamy. If it is too firm, add more motherless milk.
5. Taste and add spice if needed.

Vegetable Lentil Salad

Think of this salad as an entire meal. Just look at all the ingredients and the flavor combos and you can see how I say this is a meal all by itself.

HONEY MUSTARD DRESSING:

2 tablespoon Dijon mustard—our favorite mustard is
    Kozliks from Canada
3 tablespoons maple syrup
Juice of ½ lemon
1 small garlic clove, minced

SALAD INGREDIENTS:

1 large zucchini chopped
¼ cup vegetable broth low sodium
1 cup corn
1 cup cooked green or red lentils

2 small carrots, finely chopped
½ cup cherry tomatoes sliced in half
No-salt all-purpose seasoning and pepper

Instructions:

1. Combine Dijon, honey, lemon, and garlic in a small bowl and stir to combine. Season with pepper to taste. Set aside.
2. Heat a medium skillet over medium heat. Add zucchini and veggie broth with no-salt all-purpose seasoning and pepper to taste. Sauté until it starts to get tender (3-5 minutes). Add corn and sauté until zucchini and corn are caramelized and brown (5-7 minutes).
3. Put cooked lentils in a large bowl. Add sautéed zucchini and corn, carrots, and tomatoes. Toss with dressing to taste. Only add salt if needed after tasting.

Stuffed Pesto Mushrooms

These mushrooms will be the first to disappear at your next dinner party or pot luck. They are so easy; they don't even need an ingredient list or instructions. Just go buy any mushroom you want—cremini or button work the best—de-stem them and then stuff them full of my pesto from the recipe earlier. Heat them in a 350 F oven for 20 minutes and pow!

Vegetable Rice Stuffed Peppers

I don't know which is more my favorite, my lasagna or these stuffed peppers. I always make enough for at least two days, and actually, they taste better the second day. I usually use a variety of red, yellow, and orange peppers. The green peppers are not my favorite, but if green works for you, go for it.

4-6 peppers (red, yellow, orange)
1 cup cooked brown rice
Veggie broth, white wine, or water
1 can drained cooked black beans
1 can drained corn
1 cup mushrooms
1 large onion minced
3-4 cloves garlic minced
2-3 finely chopped carrots
2-3 stalks finely chopped celery
½ teaspoon cumin
¼ teaspoon cayenne pepper
¼ cup nutritional yeast as topping
Parsley or avocado for garnish
Cashew cheese from lasagna recipe from earlier as
    topping or mixed in.

Instructions:

1. Preheat oven to 350 F.
2. Line a baking pan with parchment paper.
3. Cup tops off peppers and take out inner parts.
4. Cook peppers upside down in oven until peppers are semi soft—about 15 minutes.

5. While the peppers are cooking, preheat frying pan with a few tablespoons veggie broth, wine, or water, and add the onion and garlic. Cook stirring constantly 3-4 minutes.

6. Add veggies and spices and cook till done.

7. Take pan off heat and add in corn, beans, and rice—mix together.

8. Stuff peppers and return to oven to cook for 30 minutes.

9. Top either with nutritional yeast, cashew cheese, parsley, and/or avocado.

Cauli-Power Vegetable Risotto

Again my good friend and fellow whole food, plant-based eater Riley Shaia shared this recipe with me. Note that this dish is enough to feed a baseball team which she does feed on a regular basis. If you don't want to cook so much, then just use ½ the amounts, but better yet, cook the recipe as is and you will have leftovers for days. Freeze some for later or share with your own baseball team.

RISOTTO

7-8 cups vegetable broth
1 large bunch asparagus
2 medium red bell peppers, thinly sliced
4 carrots, peeled and sliced
2 cups Arborio rice
½ tsp each salt and pepper
½ cup dry white wine (or sub more vegetable broth)
½ cup almond parmesan cheese (recipe above)

CHEESE SAUCE:

4 heaping cups cauliflower
1 heaping tablespoon minced garlic
½ cup unflavored plant milk
¼ nutritional yeast
1 tablespoon fresh lemon juice
½ teaspoon garlic powder
¾ teaspoon salt or to taste
½ teaspoon pepper or to taste

Instructions:

1. In a medium saucepan, heat vegetable broth over medium heat. Once simmering, reduce temperature to low to keep warm.
2. In the meantime, heat a large pan over medium heat. Add a bit of water and the peppers, asparagus, and carrots. Season with salt and pepper and sauté until tender (3-4 minutes).
3. Remove vegetables from the pan and set aside. In the same pan, add garlic and rice, cooking for 1 minute, stirring occasionally. Add white wine and stir gently, cooking for 1-2 minutes until liquid is absorbed.
4. Using a ladle, add warmed vegetable broth ½ cup at a time, stirring almost constantly. The temperature should be medium, and a slight simmer should be maintained at all times. Continue until the rice is "al dente" (cooked through but not mushy).

5. Remove from heat, season with salt and pepper, add the parmesan cheese and the cooked vegetables.
6. While the rice is cooking, steam the cauliflower in the microwave or on the stovetop until tender.
7. Place the steamed cauliflower and rest of cheese sauce in a blender and blend until smooth.
8. Season with additional salt and pepper to taste.

Bruce's Best

Tempeh Mushroom Stir Fry
Jackfruit BBQ
What Every Salad Shouldn't Go Without—Bruce's Killer Salad Dressing
Bruce's Killer Super Picker Upper Snack
Tempeh Mushroom Stir Fry

Because we want to provide ongoing resources for you, we are adding new recipes on our website all the time. We also have them transcribed so you can read the transcript as well. So, here is Bruce cooking up this stir fry in his own words.

Tempeh Mushroom Stir Fry

Today, I'm going to make one of my favorite recipes. It involves organic tempeh. It's one of the oldest, most ancient foods on the planet. It originated in Indonesia, and it's basically fermented, organic tofu.

It's high in protein, it's got a ton of nutrients in it. And because of the fermentation, it's good for your gut biome as well. I'm going to chop it up and then I'm going to marinade it overnight.

My tempeh marinade consists of the following. I use:

4 teaspoons of low-sodium vegetable broth
1 teaspoon of vegan Worcestershire sauce
1 teaspoon of reduced sodium soy sauce
1 teaspoon of fermented garlic black sauce, and
2 teaspoons of any red wine.

Mix it all together, then I squeeze in half of a lime, and then maybe half a teaspoon, I don't even measure the lemon. Just a little bit of lemon. And that's basically it.

Cut up the tempeh, chop it up very fine, and mix it into marinade and leave it in the fridge. We're going to cook it tomorrow, and it's going to be delicious.

Tempeh comes in a double plastic bag. I just cut the bag open. It's one piece, it's very similar, and has the firmness and texture of tofu—maybe little bit firmer. And what I like is, it ends up looking like ground turkey or ground pork. So I slice it very thin, and then this is all going to happen very fast.

Okay, now that I've diced up most of the tempeh, I'm going to dice it up even more when we start cooking it tomorrow after it's marinated overnight. That's basically what it's going to look like going in there, just like that.

And it's a great, wonderful substitute if you like ground turkey, ground chicken, ground pork, ground beef, whatever it is, this is a wonderful healthy substitute. Won't lock up your arteries and veins.

If you have Tupperware, then you can even shake it up. And then I'm just going to basically pop that in the fridge overnight and then tomorrow, we're going to cook it.

I marinated the tempeh overnight in the refrigerator with my marinade, which is primarily my salad dressing. We're going to open it up now. And you will see that it has soaked up almost all the marinade—all that flavor that's coming from those delicious herbs, spices, and dressings. Just gonna pop it right in there.

And now I'm going to sauté this tempeh for probably just five minutes. It doesn't really need to be cooked that long. And while I do that, I'm going to continue to chop it up. And now you can see it is actually starting to look a little bit like ground beef or ground turkey. So you can use this for tacos, anything to replace ground meat, use tempeh or tofu because you eliminate all the animal protein, all the problems that come along with that. You're leaving the world a better place too.

So we're going to sauté this for about 10 minutes and then we try it. I've been sautéing the tempeh now for only about four-five minutes. It has reduced down, and it smells delicious. You can now use this on tacos, and you can use it, if you like, like pork—you know, ground pork with string beans over the holidays, a lot of people make that. Throw tempeh in there instead.

This is ready to go. This is what I'm going to do. I have made some delicious sautéed mushrooms, it's in a video, just look at sautéed mushrooms on my website, onedaytowellness.org and you can see it. I'm going to mix some of these sautéed mushrooms in—actually I'm gonna put them all in.

Boom. So now I've got a nice combination of already cooked sautéed mushrooms mixing it with that tempeh. This will be good for two or three or four days actually, and it actually gets tastier here as it sits in your refrigerator because it marinates even more.

You can use this for just about anything. It is a wonderful transition to get off of eating disease-promoting animal products. Boom.

To actually see Bruce making this recipe go to onedaytowellness.com website.

Jackfruit BBQ

Our great friends from Tomball, TX, Will and Katie Benson, first introduced us to Jack fruit a few years ago. They had attended our full day One Day to Wellness and Cooking and Coaching programs and they were sold. They went from carnivore to herbivore in a nano second. Like us, they were divers not dippers, and every time we went to visit them they had another recipe to share. But did I mention they live in Texas? Texas is the BBQ capital of the world. If it isn't BBQ, it isn't food. Will had to find something to replace his pulled pork sliders that he was known for countywide. This is what he came up with without losing face or taste.

Jackfruit can be easily mistaken for pulled pork when seasoned properly. The look, taste, and texture resemble the best BBQ out there. Jackfruit by itself is hard to handle, so look for the canned brined jackfruit. Open the can and run the jackfruit under cool water, shredding it apart into a colander. Make this version of the traditional sliders—just call it BBQ and no one will be the wiser.

4 cloves garlic

1 onion

1 teaspoon minced ginger root

1 20-oz. can jackfruit drained and rinsed in water

½ cup veggie broth

1 tablespoon each soy sauce and hoisin sauce

2 cups shredded cabbage

1 cup shredded carrots

3-4 shallots cut up

Instructions:

1. Mix together garlic, onion, and ginger root in a pan with just enough veggie broth or water as needed to cook.

2. Add jackfruit, veggie broth, soy sauce and hoisin sauce.

3. Cook until jackfruit breaks apart and starts to shred.

4. Add cabbage, carrots, shallots and cook until done.

5. Serve over lettuce leaves or whole wheat bun with BBQ sauce to taste.

Bruce's Killer Salad Dressing

1-2 cloves garlic finely chopped
⅛ to ¼ cup balsamic vinegar
1 teaspoon white wine
The juice of ½ of a lemon
½ teaspoon Bragg Liquid Aminos or low sodium soy
     sauce

Instructions:

Add all ingredients together and then taste. Add additional spices if needed. Sometimes I will add:

Mustard
Maple syrup
Dill spice
Hot sauce
Capers

Bruce's Killer Super Picker Upper Snack

The first time Bruce made this snack for me, I hated it. Then little by little my taste buds adapted to the crazy collection of flavors, and now I crave it. This is not a concoction for the weak and fearful. This is a power pack punch that provides energy, antioxidants, and zing. Give it a try—multiple times. And I promise you that this will grow on you and will become a staple.

1 thin slice each
Turmeric
Dried ginger
Organic lemon with the rind

Instructions:

Construct like a piece of sushi. Place the lemon with rind on a plate. Stack dried ginger and then turmeric on top of lemon.

Add a little cracked pepper on top and pop entire thing into your mouth and chew thoroughly and swallow.

SNACKS / DESSERTS

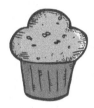

Mindy's Famous Balls (Date and Nut Ball Variations)
Roasted Chestnuts
Chocolate Mousse
Black Bean Brownies
Chickpea Cookie Dough
Oatmeal Cookies
Chocolate Pudding
Pecan Bars
Chia Pudding

Mindy's Famous Balls

I should call these "Little Mighty Energy Balls" as they are perfect as an anytime snack when you need an energy boost. Pop a couple in your mouth before a workout and wow pow. Or anytime as a tasty treat. They are our go-to snack and the base is interchangeable with lots of different ingredients to make many flavor combinations.

BASE INGREDIENTS:

½ cup walnuts
½ cup cashews (or almonds)
1 cup pitted dates
1 tablespoon vanilla
Instructions:
Mix nuts together in food processor
Then add dates and vanilla
Form into balls and freeze

BALL OPTIONS ADDITIONS

¼ cup Cacao powder
or
Cinnamon, cloves, and nutmeg
or
Coconut and chopped walnuts
or
Almond or peanut butter and cacao nips

Roasted Chestnuts

Bruce and I went to Portugal a few years ago and roasted chestnuts were sold at every street corner. We fell in love with the nutty sweet taste and thought for sure these were loaded with fat and calories. Chestnuts are full of fiber, vitamin C, and minerals like copper and potassium, and to our surprise, they are also low in fat. So, eat away.

Ingredients:

Raw chestnuts

Instructions:

1. Preheat oven to 425 degrees
2. Score the chestnut (cut an X in the center of the chestnut)
3. Line a baking sheet with parchment paper and put the chestnuts on the parchment paper with the X facing up
4. Bake at 425 until the outer shell peels back - around 15-25 minutes
5. Let cool for about 15 minutes and peel away outer shell and eat or include as a topping to soups or salads or included in stir fries

Chocolate Mousse

You will be blown away by the taste of this mousse. Every ingredient in this mousse is health promoting. No added fat, and the sugar is from dates. How wonderful is that?

Want to be sure to be invited back to the party? Bring this mousse in a pretty glass serving dish and have everyone try to guess what the ingredients are. Watch people fall on the floor when you tell them.

1 package silken tofu
2 cups date paste (1 cup water and 1 cup dates blended together to form a paste)
¼ cup cacao powder
1 teaspoon vanilla

Instructions:

1. In a blender combine paste and water and pulverize

2. Add tofu, cacao powder, and vanilla and blend until creamy

3. Chill in fridge for one hour. Good luck making it to the fridge before consuming it all.

Black Bean Brownies

These brownies are the best of the best of the best. They are moist, super delicious, and very filling. These yummy treats are also so good for you. Black beans, dates, ground flax, cacao powder, and nut butter. How much healthier can you get for a treat? I make a few batches at a time. Eat some, fridge some, and freeze some. They are a go-to when the going gets tough and you are looking for something to satisfy both your chocolatey and sweet tooth.

15 oz. can cooked black beans drained and rinsed
1½ cup date paste (1 cup pitted dates and ¾ cup warm water blended together)
¼ cup nut butter of choice
½ cup raw cacao powder
2 tablespoons ground flax seed
1 tablespoon vanilla extract
½ teaspoon baking powder
½ teaspoon baking soda (optional)
¾ cup vegan chocolate chips (optional)

Instructions:

1. Line an 8-inch square baking dish with parchment paper.
2. Blend dates and water to create paste
3. Add all additional ingredients except chocolate chips into food processor and blend until smooth.
4. Spoon chocolate chips into batter and mix together
5. Put all into parchment paper lined baking dish and cook for 20-30 minutes at 350 degrees depending on if you like a moister or drier brownie

Chickpea Cookie Dough

Every time I make these I am blown away by the dense buttery taste without the butter. Bake these for your next get together and ask the tasters what the batter is made of. Bet people for money on what it is and you will walk away with a whole lot of cash in your pocket. So not only are these delicious they will make you money.

DOUGH

1 can chickpeas, drained
½ cup nut butter of choice
¼ cup oat or other plant milk
½ cup date sugar
2 tsp vanilla
⅛ tsp baking powder

ADD INS

½ cup vegan chocolate chips
Or
½ teaspoon each clove, nutmeg, cinnamon
½ cup currants or raisins
Or
½ cup uncooked old-fashioned oatmeal
¼ cup walnuts
½ cup raisins

Instructions:

1. Preheat the oven to 350 degrees.
2. Combine all cookie dough ingredients except Extras in a bowl or high-speed blender until no more whole chickpeas remain.
3. Add chocolate chips and stir.
4. Scoop 1-inch-thick balls onto a cookie sheet lined with parchment paper or use non-stick cookie sheet. Flatten with the back of a spoon and place in the oven.
5. Bake for 15-20 minutes.
6. Remove from oven and let cool.

Oatmeal Banana Cookies

Health promoting energy releasing cookies should always fill your cookie jar. (Does anyone even own a cookie jar anymore?) Keep these cookies around for an anytime snack. They also double as a grab-and-go breakfast.

Flax egg (2 teaspoons ground flaxseed mixed with
  2 tablespoons water)
1 cup whole wheat flour (or white whole wheat)
1 cup old fashioned oats
½ teaspoon baking soda
½ teaspoon baking powder
½ teaspoon salt
1 teaspoon cinnamon
½ teaspoon vanilla
¼ cup maple syrup or date syrup
1 mashed over ripe banana
½ teaspoon lemon juice

Instructions:

1. Preheat Oven to 375 F.
2. Mix all dry then add wet ingredients.
3. Spoon onto cookie trays lined with parchment paper.
4. Cook at 375 F for 8-12 minutes.

Chocolate Fudge Pudding

I got the inspiration for this pudding from Dr. John McDougal's book, *Starch Solution,* but I didn't want to add straight-up sugar so I went to my go-to date sugar. And because I am using oat milk, that is naturally sweet, my use of sugar is less. I also usually always opt for cacao powder over cocoa powder.

Definition: "**Cacao** refers to any of the food products derived from the **cacao** bean that have remained 'raw.'

Cacao powder is known to have a higher antioxidant content than **cocoa**, and **cacao** is the purest form of chocolate you can consume, which means it is raw and much less processed than **cocoa** powder **or** chocolate bars."

> 3 cups non-dairy milk (my favorite is unsweetened oat milk)
> ½ cup cacao powder
> ¾ cup date sugar
> 1 tablespoon vanilla
> 1-3 tablespoons corn starch (add at end in small doses until pudding is the thickness you enjoy)

Instructions:

1. Cook all ingredients on medium heat on the stove stirring constantly.
2. Add corn starch after all has cooked and ingredients start to thicken. Add only enough corn starch to thicken to your liking.
3. Refrigerate for at least ½ hour before eating.

Pecan Bars

Don't make these bars unless you have a strong will and a safe that someone else has the code to and not you. I cannot make these as I will eat them all. Yes, they are that good. Just be warned. This is also from Riley Shaia. Blame her and not me.

PECAN LAYER

5-7 Medjool pitted dates
½ cup raw pecan butter

1½ cups raw pecan halves
1 tsp vanilla
¼ tsp salt (optional)

CHOCOLATE LAYER

½ cup vegan chocolate chips
¼ cup raw pecan butter

TOPPING

¼ cup chopped raw pecans

Instructions:

1. Line an 8-inch square baking dish with parchment paper.
2. Make the pecan layer by adding dates and nut butter to a food processor. Blend until you get a cohesive, sticky, crumbly mixture.
3. Add in 1 cup pecans, vanilla, and salt. Blend until the pecans are fully incorporated. It is ready when you can pinch the mixture between your fingers, and it holds together. Add in the remaining ½ cup pecans and pulse just a few times and medium-small pieces are still visible.
4. Pour this mixture into the pan and press down to create a tightly packed layer.
5. Melt the chocolate and nut butter in the microwave or on the stovetop until all the chocolate is melted. Pour over pecan layer and smooth. Add topping to the top of the bars and press down gently.
6. Freeze for 20-30 minutes then slice into 16 bars.

Chia Pudding

This pudding is not too sweet, and it has the consistency of tapioca pudding. So, if these two descriptions appeal to you, then this is your pudding. I always have to double the batch as Bruce will eat the whole bowl in one sitting.

2 cups non-dairy milk (my favorite is unsweetened oat milk)
½ cup chia seeds
1 teaspoon date syrup
1 tablespoon vanilla
½ teaspoon cinnamon

Instructions:

Mix all together and chill about 2 hours. That's it. Enjoy.

RESOURCES

Websites

American College of Lifestyle Medicine.
   https://www.lifestylemedicine.org/.

Campbell, T. Colin. "Center for Nutrition Studies."
   http://nutritionstudies.org/.

Greger, Dr. Michael. "NutritionFacts.org"
   https://nutritionfacts.org/.

Healthline. Healthline Media. http://healthline.com/.

Mylrea, Bruce and Mindy Mylrea. "One Day to Wellness."
   http://onedaytowellness.org/.

Physicians Committee for Responsible Medicine.
   https://www.pcrm.org/.

Robbins, John and Ocean. "Food Revolution Network."
   https://foodrevolution.org/.

The Plantrician Project. https://plantricianproject.org/.

---

* All sites and hyperlinks were accessed on April 7, 2020, and were live and in working order.

References (Online)

Aldemir, M. et. al. "Pistachio diet improves erectile function parameters and serum lipid profiles in patients with erectile dysfunction." International Journal of Impotence Research (IJIR) Your Sexual Medicine Journal. Jan. 13, 2011. https://www.nature.com/articles/ijir201033.

Andersen, K. V. and G. Bovim. "Impotence and Nerve Entrapment in Long Distance Amateur Cyclists." *PubMed.gov.* Apr. 1997. https://pubmed.ncbi.nlm.nih.gov/9150814/.

App - Download. "21-Day Vegan Kickstart." *Physicians Committee for Responsible Medicine.* 2020. https://kickstart.pcrm.org/en.

App - Download. "Dr. Greger's Daily Dozen." *NutritionFacts.org.* https://apps.apple.com/us/app/dr-gregers-daily-dozen/id1060700802.

Applegate, Catherine C. et. al. "Soy Consumption and the Risk of Prostate Cancer: An Updated Systematic Review and Meta-Analysis." *PubMed.gov.* Jan. 4, 2018. https://pubmed.ncbi.nlm.nih.gov/29300347/.

Azadzoi, Kazem M. et. al. "Oxidative Stress in Arteriogenic Erectile Dysfunction: Prophylactic Role of Antioxidants." *PubMed.gov.* July 2005. https://pubmed.ncbi.nlm.nih.gov/15947695/.

Bailey, Stephen J. et. al. "Dietary Nitrate Supplementation Reduces the O2 Cost of Low-Intensity Exercise and Enhances Tolerance to High-Intensity Exercise in Humans" *PubMed.gov.* Oct. 2009.
https://pubmed.ncbi.nlm.nih.gov/19661447/.

Bègue, Laurent et. al. "Some like it hot: Testosterone predicts laboratory eating behavior of spicy food." *Science Direct (Elsevier Physiology & Behavior).* Feb. 2015, Vol. 139, pg. 375-377..
https://www.sciencedirect.com/science/article/abs/pii/S0031938414005940.

Blue Zones. "The World's #1 Longevity Food."
https://www.bluezones.com/2016/06/10-things-about-beans/.

"Cacao vs Cocoa—What's the difference?" *Creative Nature.* Jan. 25, 2017.
https://www.creativenaturesuperfoods.co.uk/cacao-vs-cocoa-whats-the-difference/.

Capogrosso, Paolo et. al. "One Patient Out of Four with Newly Diagnosed Erectile Dysfunction Is a Young Man—Worrisome Picture from the Everyday Clinical Practice." *The Journal of Sexual Medicine.* July 2013. Vol. 10. 7:1833-1841.
https://onlinelibrary.wiley.com/doi/abs/10.1111/jsm.12179.

Cassidy, Aedín, Mary Franz, and Eric B. Rimm. "Dietary flavonoid intake and incidence of erectile dysfunction." *The American Journal of Clinical Nutrition.* Feb. 2016. Vol. 103, Issue 2. pg. 534-541. https://www.ncbi.nlm.nih.gov/pmc/articles/PMC4733263/.

"Chemicals in Meat Cooked at High Temperatures and Cancer Risk." NIH *National Cancer Institute.* July 11, 2017. https://www.cancer.gov/about-cancer/causes-prevention/risk/diet/cooked-meats-fact-sheet.

Cleveland Clinic. "Heart Disease & Erectile Dysfunction." *Cleveland Clinic Health Library.* July 17, 2019. https://my.clevelandclinic.org/health/diseases/15029-heart-disease--erectile-dysfunction.

Cormio, Luigi et. al. "Oral L-citrulline Supplementation Improves Erection Hardness in Men With Mild Erectile Dysfunction." *PubMed.gov.* Jan. 2011. https://pubmed.ncbi.nlm.nih.gov/21195829/.

d'Uscio, Livius V. et. al. "Long-term Vitamin C Treatment Increases Vascular Tetrahydrobiopterin Levels and Nitric Oxide Synthase Activity." *PubMed.gov.* Jan. 10, 2003. https://pubmed.ncbi.nlm.nih.gov/12522125/.

Darmadi-Blackberry, Irene et. al. "Legumes: The Most Important Dietary Predictor of Survival in Older People of Different Ethnicities." *PubMed.gov.* 2004. https://pubmed.ncbi.nlm.nih.gov/15228991/.

Das, N. S. Khan, and S. R. Sooranna. "Potent Activation of Nitric Oxide Synthase by Garlic: A Basis for Its Therapeutic Applications." *PubMed.gov.* 1995. https://pubmed.ncbi.nlm.nih.gov/7555034/.

Ekelund, Ulf. et. al. "Does physical activity attenuate, or even eliminate, the detrimental association of sitting time with mortality? A harmonised meta-analysis of data from more than 1 million men and women." *The Lancet.* Sept. 24, 2016. Vol. 388, Issue 10051, pp. 1302-1310. https://www.thelancet.com/pdfs/journals/lancet/PIIS0140-6736(16)30370-1.pdf.

Fields, Heather et. al. "Is Meat Killing Us?" *The Journal of the American Osteopathic Association.* May 2016. Vol. 116:296-300. https://jaoa.org/article.aspx?articleid=2517494.

Figueroa, Arturo et. al. "Influence of L-citrulline and Watermelon Supplementation on Vascular Function and Exercise Performance." *PubMed.gov.* Jan. 2017. https://pubmed.ncbi.nlm.nih.gov/27749691/.

Forest, C. P., H. Padma-Nathan, and H. R. Liker. "Efficacy and Safety of Pomegranate Juice on Improvement of Erectile Dysfunction in Male Patients with Mild to Moderate Erectile Dysfunction: A Randomized, Placebo-Controlled, Double-Blind, Crossover Study." *PubMed.gov.* Nov.-Dec. 2007. https://pubmed.ncbi.nlm.nih.gov/17568759/.

Fraga, César G. "Cocoa flavanols: effects on vascular nitric oxide and blood pressure." *Journal of Clinical Biochemistry and Nutrition.* 2010. Vol. 48, Issue 1, pg. 63-67.
https://www.jstage.jst.go.jp/article/jcbn/48/1/48_11-010FR/_article.

Fulgoni 3rd, Victor L., Mark Dreher, and Adrienne J. Davenort. "Avocado Consumption Is Associated with Better Diet Quality and Nutrient Intake, and Lower Metabolic Syndrome Risk in US Adults: Results From the National Health and Nutrition Examination Survey (NHANES) 2001-2008." *PubMed.gov.* Jan. 2, 2013.
https://pubmed.ncbi.nlm.nih.gov/23282226/.

GBD 2016 Alcohol Collaborators. "Alcohol use and burden for 195 countries and territories, 1990–2016: a systematic analysis for the Global Burden of Disease Study 2016." *The Lancet.* Aug. 23, 2018.
https://www.thelancet.com/journals/lancet/article/PIIS 0140-6736(18)31310-2/fulltext.

Golan, Rachel, Yftach Gepner, and Iris Shai. "Wine and Health—New Evidence." *PubMed.gov.* July 2019.
https://pubmed.ncbi.nlm.nih.gov/30487561/.

Hellmich, Nanci. "Are you sitting down? Your heart failure risk is higher." *USA Today.* Mar. 31, 2014.
https://www.usatoday.com/story/news/nation/2014/01/21/sitting-disease-heart-failure/4661431/.

Henson, J. et. al. "Associations of objectively measured sedentary behaviour and physical activity with markers of cardiometabolic health." *PubMed.gov*. May 2013. https://pubmed.ncbi.nlm.nih.gov/23456209/.

Herrington, Diana. "Pass On the Gas—7 Ways to Avoid Bean Flatulence." *Huffpost*. Nov. 28, 2019. https://www.huffingtonpost.ca/diana-herrington/pass-on-the-gas-7-ways-to_b_3080786.html.

Hightower, Jane M. and Dan Moore. "Mercury Levels in High-End Consumers of Fish." *Environmental Health Perspectives, U.S. National Library of Medicine, National Institutes of Health*. Apr. 2003. https://www.ncbi.nlm.nih.gov/pmc/articles/PMC1241452/.

Hopkins, W. G., Hawley, J. A., and L. M. Burke. "Design and Analysis of Research on Sport Performance Enhancement." *PubMed.gov*. Mar. 1999. https://pubmed.ncbi.nlm.nih.gov/10188754/.

Hurlbert, David Farley and Karen Elizabeth Whittaker. "The role of masturbation in marital and sexual satisfaction: A comparative study of female masturbators and non-masturbators." *APA PsycNET (American Psychological Association)*. 1991. https://psycnet.apa.org/record/1993-33191-001.

Inman, Brant A. et. al. "A Population-Based, Longitudinal Study of Erectile Dysfunction and Future Coronary Artery Disease." *PubMed.gov*. Feb. 2009. https://pubmed.ncbi.nlm.nih.gov/19181643/.

Kahn, Joel. "What Does Sex Have to Do with Nutrition?" *Posts Healthy Living Solutions.* Nov. 3, 2018. https://posts.rhealthylivingsolutions.com/nutrition/what-does-sex-have-to-do-with-nutrition/.

Karabakakn, M. et al. "Association Between Serum Folic Acid Level and Erectile Dysfunction". *PubMed.gov.* June 2016. https://pubmed.ncbi.nlm.nih.gov/26302884/.

Kravitz, Len. "Research Sheds New Light on the Exercise 'Afterburn.'" *IDEA Fitness Journal.* 2015. Vol. 12, Issue 4, pp. 16-18. https://www.unm.edu/~lkravitz/Article%20folder/ExerciseAfterburn2015.html.

Kroll, Juliet L. et. al. "Acute Ingestion of Beetroot Juice Increases Exhaled Nitric Oxide in Healthy Individuals." *PubMed.gov.* Jan. 25, 2018. https://pubmed.ncbi.nlm.nih.gov/29370244/.

Larson, Holly. "The Beginner's Guide to Cruciferous Vegetables." *eat right, Academy of Nutrition and Dietetics.* Feb. 21, 2018. https://www.eatright.org/food/vitamins-and-supplements/nutrient-rich-foods/the-beginners-guide-to-cruciferous-vegetables.

Le, Brian and Arthur L. Burnett. "Evolution of penile prosthetic devices." *PubMed.gov.* Mar. 3, 2015. https://www.ncbi.nlm.nih.gov/pmc/articles/PMC4355428/.

Lopez, David S. et. al. "Oral L-citrulline Supplementation Improves Erection Hardness in Men with Mild Erectile Dysfunction." *Plos One.* Apr. 28, 2015. https://journals.plos.org/plosone/article?id=10.1371/jo urnal.pone.0123547.

Lyon, France. "IARC Monographs evaluate consumption of red meat and processed meat." *Scoop Health.* Oct. 26, 2015. https://www.scoop.co.nz/stories/GE1510/S00100/iarc -evaluates-consumption-of-red-meat-and-processed- meat.htm.

Maiorino, Maria Ida, Guiseppe Bellastella, and Katherine Esposito. "Lifestyle modifications and erectile dys-function: what can be expected?" *Asian Journal of Andrology.* 2014. Vol. 17, Issue 1, pg. 5-10. http://www.ajandrology.com/article.asp?issn=1008- 682X;year=2015;volume=17;issue=1;spage=5;epage= 10;aulast=Maiorino.

Mann, Theresa N. et. al. "Effect of Exercise Intensity on Post-Exercise Oxygen Consumption and Heart Rate Recovery." *PubMed.gov.* Sep. 2014. https://pubmed.ncbi.nlm.nih.gov/24878688/.

McLeod, Saul. "Cognitive Dissonance." *Simply Psychol-ogy.* 2018. https://www.simplypsychology.org/cognitive- dissonance.html.

Menotti, A. et. al. "Food Intake Patterns and 25-year Mortality from Coronary Heart Disease: Cross-Cultural Corre-lations in the Seven Countries Study. The Seven Countries Study Research Group." *Pub.Med.gov.* July 1999. https://pubmed.ncbi.nlm.nih.gov/10485342/.

Milkowski, Andres et. al. "Nutritional Epidemiology in the context of Nitric Oxide Biology: A Risk-Benefit Evaluation for Dietary Nitrite and Nitrate." *PubMed.gov.* Feb. 15, 2010.
https://pubmed.ncbi.nlm.nih.gov/19748594/.

Mirmiran, Parvin et. al. "The Association of Dietary l-Arginine Intake and Serum Nitric Oxide Metabolites in Adults: A Population-Based Study." *MDPI.* May 20, 2016. https://www.mdpi.com/2072-6643/8/5/311.

Montorsi, Piero et. al. "The Artery Size Hypothesis: A Macrovascular Link Between Erectile Dysfunction and Coronary Artery Disease." *PubMed.gov.* Dec. 26, 2005. https://pubmed.ncbi.nlm.nih.gov/16387561/.

Multicenter Study. "Mercury, fish oils, and the risk of myocardial infarction." *PubMed.gov.* Nov. 28, 2002. https://pubmed.ncbi.nlm.nih.gov/12456850/.

Murphy, Margaret et. al. "Whole Beetroot Consumption Acutely Improves Running Performance." *PubMed.gov.* Apr. 2012. https://pubmed.ncbi.nlm.nih.gov/22709704/.

National Institutes of Health. "Coronary Artery Disease: Also called CAD, Coronary arteriosclerosis, Coronary atherosclerosis." *MedlinePlus.* Nov. 2016. https://medlineplus.gov/coronaryarterydisease.html.

Reynolds, Jeff M. and Len Kravitz. "Resistance Training and EPOC." *IDEA Personal Trainer.* 2001. Vol. 12, Issue 5, pp. 17-19.
https://www.unm.edu/~lkravitz/Article%20folder/epoc.html.

Rodriguez, Katherine M. and Alexander W. Pastuszak. "A history of penile implants." *PubMed.gov.* 2017. https://pubmed.ncbi.nlm.nih.gov/29238664/.

Saleh, Naveed. "10 natural remedies to boost virility." *MDLinx.* June 6, 2019. https://www.mdlinx.com/internal-medicine/article/3752.

Schor, Jacob. "Pistachio Nuts and Erectile Dysfunction: Snacking on pistachios improves erectile function and cardiovascular health markers." *Natural Medicine Journal.* Feb. 2012. Vol. 4, Issue 2. https://www.naturalmedicinejournal.com/journal/2012-02/pistachio-nuts-and-erectile-dysfunction.

Schrader, Steven M. et. al. "Nocturnal Penile Tumescence and Rigidity Testing in Bicycling Patrol Officers." *PubMed.gov.* Nov-Dec. 2002. https://pubmed.ncbi.nlm.nih.gov/12399541/.

Shamsa, A. et. al. "UP-3.117: Evaluation of Saffron on Male Erectile Dysfunction Initial Report (ED)." *Urology.* Oct. 1, 2009. Vol. 74, Issue 4, Supplement S331. https://www.goldjournal.net/article/S0090-4295(09)02090-1/fulltext.

Singh, Jagdish. "Folate Content in Legumes." *BioMedical Journal of Scientific & Technical Research.* Apr. 10, 2018. https://biomedres.us/pdfs/BJSTR.MS.ID.000940.pdf.

Sparling J. "Penile Erections: Shape, Angle, and Length." *PubMed.gov.* Fall 1997.
https://pubmed.ncbi.nlm.nih.gov/9292834/?from_sing le_result=Sparling+J%5BAuthor%5D+Penile+erectio ns%3A+shape%2C+angle%2C+and+length..

Spence, J. David, David J. A. Jenkins, and Jean Davignon. "Dietary cholesterol and egg yolks: not for patients at risk of vascular disease." Nov. 2010.
https://www.ncbi.nlm.nih.gov/pmc/articles/PMC2989358/.

Sudarma, Verawati, Sri Sukmaniah, and Parlindungan Siregar. "Effect of Dark Chocolate on Nitric Oxide Serum Levels and Blood Pressure in Prehypertension Subjects." *PubMed.gov.* Oct. 2011.
https://pubmed.ncbi.nlm.nih.gov/22156352/?from_sin gle_result=Sudarma+V%5BAuthor%5D.

Szalay, Jessie. "What Are Flavonoids?" *Live Science.* Oct. 20, 2015.
https://www.livescience.com/52524-flavonoids.html.

Taborelli et. al. "Fruit and Vegetables Consumption Is Directly Associated to Survival After Prostate Cancer." *PubMed.gov.* Apr. 2017.
https://academic.oup.com/ajcn/article/103/2/534/4564 750.

Toda, Noboru, Kazuhede Ayajiki, and Tomio Okamura. "Nitric oxide and penile erectile function." *Pharmacology & Therapeutics.* May 2005.
https://www.sciencedirect.com/science/article/abs/pii/ S0163725804002153?via%3Dihub.

Tuso, Philip J. et. al. "Nutritional update for physicians: plant-based diets." *PubMed.gov*. Spring 2013. https://pubmed.ncbi.nlm.nih.gov/23704846/.

U.S. Department of Agriculture. "Broccoli, cooked, boiled, drained, without salt." *USDA Agricultural Research Service*. Apr. 1, 2019, NDB Number 11091. https://fdc.nal.usda.gov/fdc-app.html#/food-details/169967/nutrients.

Uddin, S. M. Iftekhar et al. "Erectile Dysfunction as an Independent Predictor of Future Cardiovascular Events." *AHA/ASA Journals*. July 24, 2018. https://www.ahajournals.org/doi/10.1161/CIRCULAT IONAHA.118.033990.

Vasanthi, Hannah R., Subhendu Mukherjee, and Dipak K. Das. "Potential Health Benefits of Broccoli–A Chemico–Biological Overview." *PubMed.gov*. June 2009. https://pubmed.ncbi.nlm.nih.gov/19519500/.

Vella, Chantal and Len Kravitz. "Exercise After-Burn: Research Update." *IDEA Fitness Journal*. 2004. Vol. 1, Issue 5, pp. 42-47. https://www.unm.edu/~lkravitz/Article%20folder/epo carticle.html.

Vogel, R. A., M. C. Corretti, and G. D. Plotnick. "The postprandial effect of components of the Mediterranean diet on endothelial function." *PubMed.gov*. Nov. 2000. https://pubmed.ncbi.nlm.nih.gov/11079642/?from_ter m=The+postprandial+effect+of+components+of+the +Mediterranean+diet+on+endothelial+function..

Vrentzos, George E. et. al. "Diet, serum homocysteine levels and ischaemic heart disease in a Mediterranean population." *British Journal of Nutrition.* June 2004, Vol. 91, Issue 6, pp. 1013-1019.
https://www.cambridge.org/core/journals/british-journal-of-nutrition/article/diet-serum-homocysteine-levels-and-ischaemic-heart-disease-in-a-mediterranean-population/3F4D74C84CB00D86B6E0C221C47BC1BF.

Wei, Marlynn. "Yoga for better sleep." *Harvard Health Publishing, Harvard Medical School.* Oct. 5, 2018.
https://www.health.harvard.edu/blog/8753-201512048753.

Wilson, Kathryn M. et. al. "Coffee Consumption and Prostate Cancer Risk and Progression in the Health Professionals Follow-up Study." *Journal of the National Cancer Institute (JNCI).* May 17, 2011.
https://academic.oup.com/jnci/article/103/11/876/2516503.

Wood, Angela M. et. al. "Risk thresholds for alcohol consumption: combined analysis of individual-participant data for 599 912 current drinkers in 83 prospective studies." *The Lancet.* Apr. 14, 2018.
https://www.thelancet.com/journals/lancet/article/PIIS0140-6736(18)30134-X/fulltext.

Zhao, Binghao et. al. "Erectile Dysfunction Predicts Cardiovascular Events as an Independent Risk Factor: A Systematic Review and Meta-Analysis." *The Journal of Sexual Medicine.* July 2019. Vol. 16, Issue 7:1005-1017. https://pubmed.ncbi.nlm.nih.gov/31104857/.

Zhong, Victor W. et. al. "Associations of Dietary Cholesterol or Egg Consumption with Incident Cardiovascular Disease and Mortality." *PubMed.gov*. Mar.
19, 2019.
https://pubmed.ncbi.nlm.nih.gov/30874756/.

Books

Agus, David B. *The End of Illness*. New York: Simon &
Schuster, 2012.

Barnard, Neal D. *Power Foods for the Brain: An Effective
3-Step Plan to Protect Your Mind and Strengthen
Your Memory*. Grand Central Life & Style, 2013.

Barnard, Neal D. *The Cheese Trap: How Breaking a
Surprising Addiction Will Help You Lose Weight,
Gain Energy, and Get Healthy*. Grand Central Life &
Style or Hachette, UK, 2017.

Buettner, Dan. *The Blue Zones Kitchen: 100 Recipes to Live
to 100*. Washington: National Geographic Books, 2019.

Buettner, Dan. *The Blue Zones of Happiness: Lessons from
the World's Happiest People*. Washington: National
Geographic Books, 2017.

Buettner, Dan. *The Blue Zones Solution: Eating and Living
Like the World's Healthiest People*. Washington:
National Geographic Books, 2010.

Buettner, Dan. *The Blue Zones: Lessons for Living Longer
from the People Who've Lived the Longest*. Washington:
National Geographic Books, 2010.

Campbell, T. C., and Howard Jacobson. *Whole: Rethinking the Science of Nutrition.* BenBella Books, 2013.

Campbell, T. C., and Thomas M. II. *The China Study: Revised and Expanded Edition: The Most Comprehensive Study of Nutrition Ever Conducted and the Startling Implications for Diet, Weight Loss, and Long-Term Health.* BenBella Books, 2016.

Chef AJ and Glen Merzer. *The Secrets to Ultimate Weight Loss: A revolutionary approach to conquer cravings, overcome food addiction, and lose weight without going hungry.* CreateSpace Independent Publishing Platform, May 11, 2018.

Esselstyn, Ann C., and Jane Esselstyn. *The Prevent and Reverse Heart Disease Cookbook: Over 125 Delicious, Life-Changing, Plant-Based Recipes.* London: Penguin, 2014.

Fuhrman, Joel. Super Immunity: *The Essential Nutrition Guide for Boosting Your Body's Defenses to Live Longer, Stronger, and Disease Free.* New York: HarperCollins, 2011.

Garth Davis, M.D., and Howard Jacobson. *Proteinaholic: How Our Obsession with Meat Is Killing Us and What We Can Do About It.* New York: HarperCollins or HarperOne, 2015.

Greger, Michael, and Gene Stone. *How Not to Die: Discover the Foods Scientifically Proven to Prevent and Reverse Disease.* New York: Flatiron Books, 2015.

Greger, Michael. *How Not to Diet: The Groundbreaking Science of Healthy, Permanent Weight Loss*. New York: Flatiron Books, 2019.

Greger, Michael. *The How Not to Die Cookbook: 120 Recipes Scientifically Proven to Prevent and Reverse Disease*. London: Macmillan, 2017.

Hanh, Thich N. *Fear: Essential Wisdom for Getting Through the Storm*. New York: HarperCollins or Random House, 2012.

Hever, Julieanna. *The Complete Idiot's Guide to Plant-Based Nutrition*. London: Penguin or Alpha, 2011.

Keon, Joseph. *Whitewash: The Disturbing Truth About Cow's Milk and Your Health*. Gabriola Island: New Society Publishers, 2010.

Lisle, Douglas J., and Alan Goldhamer. *The Pleasure Trap: Mastering the Force that Undermines Health & Happiness*. Book Publishing Company, 2007.

McDougall, John, and Mary McDougall. *The Starch Solution: Eat the Foods You Love, Regain Your Health, and Lose the Weight for Good!* Rodale Books, 2013.

Moss, Michael. *Salt Sugar Fat: How the Food Giants Hooked Us*. Signal, 2013.

Ornish, Dean, and Anne Ornish. *Undo It!: How Simple Lifestyle Changes Can Reverse the Onset of Most Chronic Diseases*. New York: Ballantine Books, 2019.

Pollan, Michael. *In Defense of Food: The Myth of Nutrition and the Pleasures of Eating.* London: Penguin, 2009.

Pulde, Alona, and Matthew Lederman. *Keep It Simple, Keep It Whole: Your Guide to Optimum Health.* Exsalus Health & Wellness Center, 2019.

Robbins, John. *No Happy Cows: Dispatches from the Frontlines of the Food Revolution.* Berkeley: Conari Press, 2012.

Stone, Gene. *Forks Over Knives: The Plant-Based Way to Health.* The Experiment or Penguin Group Australia, 2011.

Movies / Documentaries

Andersen, Kip and Keegan Kuhn. *Cowspiracy: The Sustainability Secret.* 2014. You Tube Video, 1:29:33. https://www.dailymotion.com/video/x2zuhks.

Anderson, Kip and Keegan Kuhn. *What the Health.* 2017. YouTube Video. 1:06:56. https://www.youtube.com/watch?v=g7kh8tLz5fs.

Cameron, James et. al. *The Game Changers.* Sep. 30, 2019. YouTube Video. 1:25:47. *https://www.youtube.com/watch?v=2E_K86jtE58.*

Chester, John and Sandra Keats. *The Big Biggest Little Farm.* Dec. 23, 2019. YouTube Video. 2:10. https://www.youtube.com/watch?v=ShYCjp1WWXY.

Fulkerson, Lee. *Forks Over Knives.* 2011. YouTube Video. 1:51:45.
https://www.youtube.com/watch?v=ij1r27_dHk0.

Greger, Michael. *Survival of the Firmest: Erectile Dysfunction & Death.* August 19, 2013. YouTube Video. 4:32. Volume 14.
https://nutritionfacts.org/video/survival-of-the-firmest-erectile-dysfunction-and-death/.

Kenner, Robert. *The Truth About Your Food with FOOD, INC.* July 17, 2012. YouTube Video 58:19.
https://www.youtube.com/watch?v=2Oq24hITFTY.

Lee Fulkerson. *Forks Over Knives.* 2011. YouTube Video. 1:51:45.
https://www.youtube.com/watch?v=ij1r27_dHk0.

Spurlock, Morgan. *Super Size Me.* 2004. YouTube Video. 1:38.41.
https://www.youtube.com/watch?v=zKQGAv8gtBA&t=40s.

ABOUT THE AUTHOR

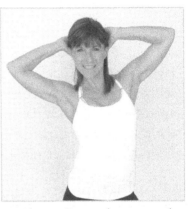

What don't you know about me by now? I didn't start out wanting to write a book based on the penis. My early passion was acting. I wanted to play Peter Pan on Broadway. I did some semiprofessional theater in my early 20s, but to pay the bills, I taught fitness. As it turned out, I was better at that than acting so fitness turned into my full-time gig. Back then I also met and married Bruce, and we went on to have three boys—Drew, Chris, and Casey. After winning the National and World Aerobic Championship in 1991, I joined the speaking circuit and now educate all over the world. I starred in my first direct response commercial, "The 6 second Abs," in the early 2000s. Shortly after that I launched the Gliding Discs for which I own two patents. The Tabata Bootcamp came next with Fluid Strength, and this year, I am co-launching a new HIIT program called "Extreme HIIT Chaos." I have starred in over 500 videos because frankly, starring in a video is so much easier than writing a book, although I authored numerous fitness and wellness articles.

It wasn't though until around 2010 that I connected the relationship between food and wellness. When Bruce was diagnosed with cancer, our entire life shifted. Fitness, as a career, wasn't the most important piece to me anymore. Nutritional education was. And the misunderstanding about this relationship is what has triggered both Bruce and I to shift our focus and create our nonprofit foundation, One Day to Wellness. There are so many people who just settle for the status quo when they personally can do so much to support their health if they only knew how. It is our job to help people understand the benefit of eating healthy, being mindful, and finding a purpose.

So this is me. A Whole Food, Plant-Based advocate educator who came up with a great name for a book. The title had to be used, and the book had to be written. I hope you enjoyed it. Thanks for reading. Now it is your turn to be the advocate and pass on the message that, with a small amount of effort, we, and our private parts, can thrive.

I will now go back to lecturing on fitness and wellness. I have added "The Plant Powered Penis" lecture to my repertoire, so I hope to see you in one or many of my lectures on the road.

ALSO AVAILABLE ON AMAZON
BRUCE'S BOOK

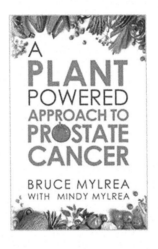

https://www.amazon.com/Plant-Powered-Approach-Prostate-Cancer/dp/B08BW8L1VG/ref=sr_1_1?crid=2KWWG4ZIV2 3CR&dchild=1&keywords=a+plant+powered+approach+to+ prostate+cancer+bruce+mylrea&qid=1596667204&sprefix=a +plant+powered%2Caps%2C188&sr=8-1

REVIEWS

Prostate cancer is one of the most common cancers in men, but that doesn't mean steps can't be taken to lower your risk. That's where nutrition comes in. A plant-based diet not only provides protection against the disease; breakthrough research shows that it can slow or even halt its progression. In this powerful book, Bruce shares his inspiring journey along with everything you need to know to regain your health.

Neal D. Barnard, MD, FACC
Adjunct Professor, George Washington
University School of Medicine
President, Physicians Committee

ARE YOU READY to take back your POWER? Bruce's inspiring story will GET YOU THERE!

I've health coached hundreds of men over a decade now, and they need this book NOW more than ever!

This book is a quick guide for any man that is dealing with Prostate Cancer! It's also a great resource for *all* Health Practitioners to share with their patients!

Michelle Joy Kramer
Board Certified Health Coach, CHHC, AADP
MichelleJoyKramer.com

This book a must-read for anyone touched by prostate cancer. Bruce reveals with honesty and humor how he leveraged his knowledge of, and passion for, plant-based nutrition, mindfulness, and personal behavioral change strategies not only to help heal himself but also to shine a light of wisdom and hope for others.

Ocean Robbins
CEO, Food Revolution Network
Author, 31-Day Food Revolution

Bruce details his remarkable journey in managing his life with a prostate cancer diagnosis. I was especially impressed with the level of engagement that Bruce made with the research community in order to ensure the accuracy of his writing.

Theodore M. Brasky, Ph.D.
Research Assistant Professor,
Dept. Internal Medicine
Ohio State University Comprehensive
Cancer Center

What a refreshing, honest account! The author and his wife Mindy use everyday language to describe his journey with cancer. He lets it all out—whatever he thinks, with additional, care-giving comments from Mindy. Bruce reveals the tight linear connection between long term dietary patterns and cancer development, then goes on to outline how we can leverage simple behavior change strategies to substantially improve cancer outcomes.

T Colin Campbell, PhD
Jacob Gould Schurman Professor
Emeritus of Nutritional Biochemistry
Cornell University

Made in USA - Kendallville, IN
55023_9798635020142
04.13.2022 1055